ESSENTIALS OF FLUID BALANCE

TO MOLLIE

'Brevity makes counsell more portable for
memorie and readier for use'

Joseph Hall, *Characters of Virtues and Vices*, 1608

'Each of us finds lucidity only in those ideas
which are in the same state of
confusion as his own'

Marcel Proust, *Within a Budding Grove*, 1918

ESSENTIALS OF FLUID BALANCE

D. A. K. BLACK

M.D. F.R.C.P.

Professor of Medicine
University of Manchester

FOURTH EDITION

SECOND PRINTING

BLACKWELL SCIENTIFIC PUBLICATIONS
OXFORD AND EDINBURGH

SBN: 632 00420 7

FIRST EDITION FEBRUARY 1957
SECOND EDITION JANUARY 1960
THIRD EDITION 1964
FOURTH EDITION 1967
SECOND PRINTING 1969

Printed by offset in Great Britain by Alden & Mowbray Ltd
at the Alden Press, Oxford
and bound at Kemp Hall Bindery

CONTENTS

INTRODUCTION, TERMINOLOGY   vii–ix

I   GENERAL PROPERTIES OF BODY-FLUID   1–18

Total body-water   1
Distribution of body-fluid   3
Electrolyte structure of the phases of body-fluid   7
Biological role of electrolytes   14

II   WATER   19–38

Thirst   19
Urinary concentration and dilution   21
Polyuria   25
Water depletion   28
Water intoxication   34

III   SODIUM   39–73

Amount and distribution   39
Sodium homeostasis   40
Sodium depletion   49
Hyponatraemic syndromes   56
Sodium excess   60

IV   POTASSIUM   74–104

Amount and distribution   74
Potassium homeostasis   76
Hypokalaemia   83
Potassium depletion   86
Clinical potassium depletion   89
Hyperkalaemia   98

v HYDRION   105–131

Hydrion homeostasis   108
'Acidosis': hydrion-excess   111
'Alkalosis': hydrion deficit   122
Relation to other disorders of body-fluid   128

vi AN APPROACH TO TREATMENT   132–150

History and examination   135
Laboratory investigations   139
Principles of Treatment   145

REFERENCES   151

INDEX   178

FIGURES

1.1 Body composition   6
1.2 Electrolyte structure of body-fluid   11
2.1 Renal actions of A.D.H.   23
2.2 Effects of sodium and of water depletion   29
3.1 Filtered and excreted water and solutes   43
4.1 Na and K in E.C.F. and I.C.F.   76
4.2 Electrocardiogram in hyperkalaemia   102
5.1 P_{CO_2}, $[HCO_3]$ and $[H]$ in blood   111

INTRODUCTION

In the past I have had the opportunity of reading, and in some cases reviewing, at least a dozen small books on the subject which I have chosen. In spite of this experience, I now find myself adding another to the pile; this exorbitant procedure can be justified, if at all, only by a clear statement of my aims in writing it, and some indication of those for whom it is written.

My first aim is to keep this book as short as possible, consistent with clarity. In order to achieve this, I have sacrificed to some extent the literature, the kidney and the details of fluid therapy. In dealing with the literature, reference has been made only to review articles and to some recent papers. Comprehensive treatment of the literature in this whole field is now impossible, except perhaps in a multiple-author book; for example, Selkurt (1954) gave 409 references in reviewing sodium excretion by the mammalian kidney and these could no doubt be doubled from the intervening decade. In this book the kidney is considered only as it influences or is influenced by the overall balance of water and electrolytes; general renal problems are discussed in Homer Smith (1951) (with 2300 references) and in a recent multiple-author book (Black, 1967). Details of the various electrolyte replacement solutions, routes of administration, and quantitative formulae for assessing deficits have also been omitted or cursorily dealt with; this has been done in the belief that principles are more important than details, and that the appearance of authenticity offered by detailed case reports is illusory, since every patient with fluid imbalance is different from every other.

My second aim, also linked to brevity, has been to make the presentation somewhat general, or—to use a word which has become rather unworthily tarnished—'academic'. Paradoxically, this means that I am appealing not to an audience of experts, but to the general medical reader, including the undergraduate. The study of electrolytes can engross a lifetime of research, but it is also much too important to be left to the specialist; and the practising doctor, who might be repelled by the details, may yet find it worth his while to read a short account of current thinking on this subject. There are now few branches of medicine or surgery in which attention to fluid and electrolyte balance cannot make some contribution to the patient's comfort, and on occasions to his survival; yet in the press of competing disciplines a work of modest proportions may gain some attention where a fuller account would be simply neglected.

The pursuit of these aims compels a certain standing back from the arena where the battles of electrolyte studies are being fought. By doing so, I may well incur the censure of the expert for over-simplification, and of the practical man for refusing to supply a numerical sign to guide treatment. I can only hope that this book may be of use to those whose main concern lies elsewhere, and that the references, while limited in number, may serve as a guide to further reading for those who find this account inadequate.

The scope of this discussion, besides water itself, extends to those electrolytes which are present in some phase of body-fluid in sufficient amount to be quantitatively important in defining osmotic or electrostatic equilibrium. These 'bulk electrolytes' of body-fluid include sodium, potassium, magnesium, and the accompanying anions chloride and bicarbonate. Within the cells, protein and phosphate make up a very considerable amount of the anions, but I have excluded them from full consideration because their proper treatment would demand an extended account of biochemical energetics and nitrogen metabolism. For similar reasons, the mineral constituents of bone have not been dealt with.

In much of the discussion, we will be concerned with the osmotic activity of electrolytes, which depends on the number of particles present in unit volume; and with the electrostatic activity, which depends on the number of charged ions. For both these purposes, it will be simpler to use a terminology which eliminates the irrelevance in this context of the different atomic weights of the different electrolytes, and gives a figure which is directly related to the number of ions. The accepted unit is the number of milliequivalents per litre (mEq/l.). Values expressed in mg/100 ml are converted to mEq/l. by multiplying by 10 (to change '100 ml' to 'a litre'), and dividing by the equivalent weight of the particular ion (to change 'mg' into 'mEq'). After this arithmetical note, it may be germane to mention that these exercises are a necessary step in bringing out the relationships between the different electrolytes only if they have been reported in W/V terminology; but it is just as easy for the clinical chemist to report electrolytes in mEq/l., and fortunately this is now generally done.

The following abbreviations have also been used:

Na	sodium
K	potassium
HCO$_3$	bicarbonate
(and other conventional chemical abbreviations)	
mEq/l.	milli-equivalents per litre
μEq/l.	micro-equivalents per litre
mμEq/l.	milli-micro-equivalents per litre *or* nano-equivalents per litre
mM/l.	millimols (or milli-osmols) per litre
E.C.G.	electrocardiogram
N.F.	National Formulary
E.C.F.	extracellular fluid
I.C.F.	intracellular fluid
G.F.R.	glomerular filtration rate
C$_x$	clearance of X
A.D.H.	pituitary anti-diuretic hormone
DCA	desoxycorticosterone acetate
ATP	adenosine tri-phosphate

Concentrations are expressed by enclosing a symbol in square brackets, e.g. [K]. The subscripts 'e' and 'i' indicate extracellular and intracellular location, e.g. [K]$_i$ is intracellular potassium concentration. *Total amounts* are given in round brackets, e.g. (K); i.e. (K) = [K] × V. *Isotopes* other than the predominant natural isotope are distinguished by a superscription before the symbol, e.g. ^{42}K.

CHAPTER I

GENERAL PROPERTIES OF BODY-FLUID

Total Body-water

Changes in the amount of water in the body can be calculated from observed changes in body-weight, after correction for food intake and excreta and the carbon lost as CO_2 in the expired air; the calculation of insensible water loss from 'insensible weight loss' is detailed by Newburgh and Johnston (1942). Very rapid changes in weight usually imply changes in fluid balance; changes in body-fat and in lean tissue mass manifest themselves more gradually.* Change in body-fluid can also be assessed with rather less accuracy by comparing the measured fluid intake and output, and correcting the intake for water derived from the oxidation of foods, and the output for insensible losses of water by skin and lungs. The water of oxidation of a normal diet is about 300 ml, and about 1000 ml of water is lost by skin and lungs, so a somewhat arbitrary correction of 700 ml may be added to the measured output before balancing it against the intake. In the presence of fever or visible sweating, the insensible water loss may rise to two litres or more per day.

The absolute amount of water in the body can be assessed by determining the volume of distribution of a substance which becomes evenly diffused through body-water. Urea, thiourea, antipyrine,

---

* An important exception to this generalization is the very rapid breakdown of fat, and to a less extent of lean tissue, which forms part of the metabolic response to injury. Moore *et al* (1952) have obtained evidence that the loss of fat after surgery or in acute severe illness may reach 600 g/day; while the loss of lean tissue is of the order of 200 g/day. This exception obviously concerns only rapid weight *loss*; gains of solid tissue of comparable rapidity have not been observed.

I

deuterium and tritium have been used in this way. The method with urea presents fewest analytical difficulties, but inaccuracy can arise from changes in the rate of urea production within the body. The deuterium oxide (heavy water) method presents more technical difficulties, but is freer from biological sources of error. Extensive studies with deuterium are reported by Edelman *et al* (1952): their results in young normal subjects can be tabulated as follows:

	No. of subjects	Age range	Body-water (as % of weight) Mean	Range
Men	34	17–34	61.1	53.3–70.3
Women	18	20–31	51.2	45.6–59.9

The results with tritium on a smaller series of normal men are similar; tritium and deuterium spaces are equal, and both are greater than the antipyrin space, a difference attributed to exchange of ^{2}H or ^{3}H with labile H in body-protein (Prentice *et al*, 1952).

From an analysis of published figures, Widdowson and Dickerson (1964) give the percentages of body-water/body-weight in men and women respectively as 59.1 and 51.0 (deuterium method); and 53.4 and 43.4 (antipyrine method).

In infants under a month, 77 per cent of the body-weight is water, and the percentage of water falls through childhood to about 60 per cent at the age of 16. In childhood, there is little difference in the water content of the sexes, but at puberty the sex difference shown in the table begins to appear. There is a further fall in the percentage of water in the body with advancing age, the lower percentage of water in women persisting. There is an inverse relationship between the percentage of water in the body and the calculated fat content of the body—a relationship which goes far to account for the lower body-water of adult women by comparison with men.

The 'body-water' which is measured by these methods has for the most part formed a gel with the protein and mucopolysaccharide of body-fluid, although collections of physical fluid are found in a few situations in the normal body, and more widely when an increase in the water content of the body has led to oedema or serious effusions. Gel formation, clearly evident in protoplasm, and probable in the extra-cellular spaces, offers no barrier to the passage of ions and small molecules, but the diffusion of larger molecules such as inulin may be delayed.

Distribution of Body-fluid

The outstanding functional division of body-fluid is into extracellular fluid and intracellular fluid, which are separated from one another by the aggregate of cell walls. The spaces occupied by these fluids are often described as 'compartments', but this term obscures an important difference of distribution, which is well brought out in an alternative diagrammatic concept of Robinson and McCance (1952). They liken E.C.F. to the continuous phase, and I.C.F. to the disperse phase of an emulsion; and this analogy emphasizes the function of E.C.F. as a transport medium penetrating all tissues, whereas the separation of I.C.F. in cells provides the anatomical basis for differentiation of cellular chemical function. We owe to Claude Bernard the apprehension that E.C.F. provided an internal environment of virtual constancy in which the tissue cells might safely graze. It is only by such an arrangement that the body can digest the tissue of other animals, or form an acid urine, without its own cells being damaged.

Extracellular fluid is rather obviously separable into intravascular and extravascular moieties, divided anatomically by vessel walls. The equilibrium between these two portions of E.C.F. is determined by the balance between on the one hand the capillary hydrostatic pressure and on the other the net colloid osmotic pressure of protein-rich plasma versus protein-poor interstitial fluid (Starling, 1909). Isotope studies have shown that interchange of ions and small molecules between plasma and interstitial fluid takes place with extreme rapidity; so it is scarcely surprising to find that these two phases of body-fluid, however anatomically discrete, are physiologically continuous in respect of their electrolyte composition.* It is also apparent that a fall in plasma volume can arise either as part of a

* Because of the protein content of plasma, there are small differences in electrolyte concentration between plasma and transudates, determined by the Donnan equilibrium and the lower percentage of water in plasma. Smith (1951) gives the following ratios:

	[Na]	[K]	[Cl]	[HCO$_3$]
E.C.F./plasma ratio	0.95	0.9	1.02	1.02

general diminution in total E.C.F. volume, or from a lack of plasma protein, which allows too high a proportion of the E.C.F. to be extravascular.

In addition to the obvious and long-established division of E.C.F. into the *plasma* compartment and the *interstitial-and-lymphatic* compartment, we are now aware of other important compartments containing fluid with the electrolyte pattern of E.C.F. These include the 'fluid' in *dense connective tissue and cartilage*; the 'fluid' in *bone*; and the collective compartment of '*transcellular fluids*', i.e. these fluids which have been secreted through cells into such spaces as the lumen of the alimentary tract or the subarachnoic space (Edelman and Leibman, 1959).

Methods are available for measuring the volume of the plasma and of the total E.C.F. There is no direct method of measuring I.C.F. volume, which can be assessed only by the difference between total body-water and E.C.F. Plasma volume is measured by determining the early volume of distribution of a substance which becomes bound to plasma protein and so does not leave the circulation rapidly; vital red, Evan's blue (T 1824) and ^{131}I have been used. The largest number of results have been obtained with T 1824; Edelman and Leibman (1959) give a mean value of 45.2 ml/kg in 69 men aged 17–39; and 43.8 ml/kg in 76 women in the same age-range.

For the measurement of total E.C.F., a substance is required which distributes itself through E.C.F., but does not enter cells; equilibration should be fairly rapid, so that urinary loss and metabolic destruction do not demand too large a correction.

The substances which have been used fall into two main groups, as is apparent from the figures collected by Widdowson and Dickerson (1964). Inulin, mannitol and thiosulphate give mean values of 15.6, 16.6, and 16.3 per cent of body-weight; whereas bromine, [38]Cl, and [24]Na give mean values of 28.4, 26.8, and 26.2 per cent. Thiocyanate, which is known to enter red cells, gives the intermediate value of 22.9 per cent. The obvious inference is that the small ions are entering tissues and fluids from which inulin, mannitol, and thiosulphate are wholly or partly excluded. Inulin does not enter C.S.F., or the fluid in the gut; and the small ions no doubt penetrate the E.C.F. of bone, cartilage, and tendon more readily. Indeed, it has been observed that tendon contains two phases of E.C.F., one rapidly penetrated by both chloride and inulin, the other (and larger) penetrated rapidly by chloride, but much more slowly by inulin (Nicholls *et al.*, 1953).

The volume of E.C.F. is somewhat lower in women than in men. In infants it is very much higher than in adults, and represents a higher proportion of their increased total body-water.

By failing to include slowly-equilibrating sectors of fluid of E.C.F. pattern, the older methods underestimated E.C.F., and so led to an over-estimate of I.C.F. Current estimates for a young man of 70 kg would work out as follows:

	% of body-weight	Litres
Plasma	4	2.8
Rapidly-equilibrating interstitial fluids	13	9.1
Slowly-equilibrating interstitial fluids	8	5.6
Transcellular fluids	2	1.4
Total E.C.F.	27	18.9
I.C.F. (by difference)	33	23.1
Total body-water	60	42.0

The different components of body-fluid have been described in some detail, because they are relevant not only to body-fluid itself (Edelman and Leibman, 1959), but also to the description of body-composition in general terms (McCance and Widdowson, 1951). Most of the variations in body-composition are due to variations in the fat and fluid components; and the 'cell mass' is itself sufficiently homogeneous to allow its calculation from cell-water. Given knowledge of the cell mass, the E.C.F. and the mineral content of the bones, the amount of fat in the body can be determined by difference; the results agree fairly well with estimates based on the specific gravity of the body.* Some of the possible applications of this

* Lean tissue can also be assessed from the total amount of ^{40}K in the body, and the results in young subjects agree well with those based on specific gravity; but in older subjects the ^{40}K method gives lower values, and thus higher estimates of fat. Myhre and Kessler (1966) suggest that this discrepancy is due to a relative preponderance in older people of 'potassium-poor' protein (connective tissue) over 'potassium-rich' protein (muscle).

technique in nutrition and in clinical medicine have been discussed by
McCance (1953), and by Hamwi and Urbach (1953). The important

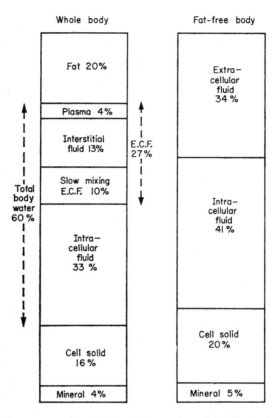

FIG. 1.1. Contribution of the different phases of body-fluid to the
mass of the whole body, and of the 'fat-free body', which is less
variable in composition.

changes which take place during growth are reviewed by Widdowson and Dickerson (1964). In Fig. 1.1, the probable composition of the
body of a young man is shown in terms of the main divisions of
body-fluid, and the amount of fat, bone mineral and the remainder,
which consists of cell solids other than fat; this remainder must
consist largely of protein, and it is interesting to note how closely

it agrees with the figure of 19/100 g given by McCance and Widdowson (1951) for the protein content of fat-free adult human tissue.

Electrolyte Structure of the Phases of Body-fluid

The electrolyte structure of E.C.F. can be determined in normal and abnormal states by analysis of plasma or serum, and the results are representative of E.C.F. in most tissues. The composition of intracellular fluid is more difficult to ascertain, because in the nature of things I.C.F. can never be obtained without admixture with E.C.F.— except in washed haemocytes, which have been useful in many studies of cation transport, but cannot be accepted as representative of the composition of body-cells in general. Moreover, the segregation of I.C.F. into separate cells, each containing subcellular particles of great complexity, makes I.C.F. something of a statistical concept rather than a samplable biological reality. There is the further problem of a reference standard: the primary measurements are (1) the weight of the tissue sample, which will include varying amounts of water, of fat, and of protein, some of which is extracellular collagen; and (2) the quantity of the different electrolytes in the sample. These primary results are simply expressed as mEq/kg of wet tissue, and even from results so expressed it is immediately obvious that whole tissue contains much more K, Mg and P, and much less Na and Cl than plasma. For example, Table 1.1 gives the mean results of Litchfield and Gaddie (1958) for 23 human muscle biopsies, and serum from the same patients.

Since at least a third of the fluid in tissue is E.C.F., it is clear that a straightforward comparison of the analysis of plasma and of tissue will not directly expose the difference in composition between E.C.F. and I.C.F. In order to arrive at the composition of I.C.F., it is necessary to calculate how much of the water in the tissue is extracellular, and also to subtract extracellular from total tissue electrolyte. Most such calculations assume that tissue Cl is entirely, or almost entirely, extracellular, though there is some evidence (Dean *et al*, 1952) that the cell wall is not the complete barrier to the Cl ion which it was once thought to be. However, the error so introduced

B

is not a large one, and it appears to be relatively constant (Manery, 1954). The content of Cl in the sample is divided by the [Cl] of E.C.F., to give a calculated E.C.F. volume, or mass; and the I.C.F. volume, or mass, is then derived by subtraction from the total. For the electrolytes other than chloride, their extracellular moiety is calculated from the E.C.F. volume in the sample, and from the concentration of that electrolyte in E.C.F.; total I.C.F. electrolyte is

TABLE 1.1

Water and electrolyte content of serum and fat-free whole muscle (man)

	Water (g/kg)	Na (mEq)	K (mEq)	Cl (mEq)
Serum (litre)	916	142	4.5	105
Muscle (kg)	772	32	102	18.5

The electrolyte results are related to a litre of serum, and to a kilogramme of fresh de-fatted muscle.

again derived by difference, and related to calculated I.C.F. volume, i.e. as mEq of electrolyte/litre of I.C.F. This is a suitable unit for comparison of E.C.F. and I.C.F. electrolyte concentrations; but it has the disadvantage that the numerical value obtained will be altered not only by changes in the electrolyte content of the tissue, but also by changes in the water content. To obviate this, we can use a reference base derived from tissue solids, so that the hydration of the tissue will not influence the numerical value obtained; it is for this reason that in different papers we find electrolyte concentrations referred to such different quantities as '100 g fat-free solids', total N, total P, non-collagen nitrogen (N.C.N.) or deoxyribonucleic-acid-phosphate (DNAP). For a fuller discussion of reference bases for tissue electrolytes, see Barnes et al (1957). In summary, the primary results are expressed in mEq/kg of fresh tissue, or mEq/kg of fat-free tissue: calculated values for I.C.F. are expressed in mEq/l. of I.C.F.

when the osmolality of I.C.F. is the main matter to be considered; but in mEq/100 g fat-free solids (or another 'dry' unit, such as N.C.N.) when there is a need to eliminate the effect of changes in

TABLE 1.2

Electrolyte structure of plasma and intracellular fluid

	Plasma mEq/l.	I.C.F mEq/kg intracellular water
Cations		
Na	142	11
K	4.5	164
Ca	5	2
Mg	3	28
Anions		
Cl	103	—
HCO_3	27	10
PO_4	2	105
SO_4	1	20
Protein	16	65
Organic acids	6	5

Based on the results of Litchfield and Gaddie (1958), and on the literature. At pH values around 7, proteins have an excess of anionic valences. The values for intracellular anions are speculative in the absence of precise knowledge of intracellular pH, and the state of intracellular CO_2 and phosphorus.

water-content. For example, a true increase in the Na content of muscle, apparent in terms of dry-weight, would be concealed by a concomitant and greater increase in water-content, if a 'wet' reference-unit were used.

For our present purpose, the general comparison of E.C.F. and I.C.F. electrolyte structure, it is sufficient to consider plasma values in mEq/l. and calculated I.C.F. values in mEq/kg of intracellular water. The values shown in Table 1.2 and Fig. 1.2 are based in part on the results of Litchfield and Gaddie (1958) on human muscle, supplemented by average values from the literature.*

The fluid outside the cells is obviously very different in its electrolyte structure from that within them. Most conspicuously, the E.C.F. is a 'sodium' fluid, while I.C.F. is a 'potassium' fluid—yet the cell wall is readily permeable both to Na and to K. The striking gradient of [Na], and of [K], across the cell-wall is contingent on the integrity of cell metabolism: but it is not known whether this dependence arises because energy is needed to run a 'sodium pump', extruding Na from the cell (Dean, 1941); or because energy is needed merely to maintain cellular organization such that anionic sites are accessible to the smaller hydrated K ion, but not to the larger hydrated Na ion (Ling, 1952). This special case of the gradient across the cell-wall has been reviewed in the general context of ion transport by Koefoed-Johnson and Ussing (1960), Cort (1963a), and Skou (1965).

The description of body-fluid must take account of certain similarities as well as the more obvious differences between E.C.F. and I.C.F.

(i) In both fluids, the cation and anion concentrations, when expressed in mEq/l., balance one another on the scale used. In other

---

* Average values like these do not of course meet the practical need for defining a normal range; this particularly affects plasma, on which routine electrolyte estimations are usually made. Wootton and King (1953) have shown that the normal values of some electrolytes, e.g. plasma potassium, are not distributed around the mean in the 'normal' or Gaussian distribution, so that the 'normal range' is not defined by the mean and standard deviation, but must be expressed as the range which excludes a predetermined percentage of results at each end. Their results for [Na], [K], [Cl] and [HCO$_3$], based on 50–100 samples of plasma from normal subjects, are as follows:

	Excluding			
	Lower 1%	Lower 10%	Upper 10%	Upper 1%
[Na] mEq/l.	133	137	148	152
[K] mEq/l.	3.5	3.9	5.0	5.6
[Cl] mEq/l.	99	101	106	108
[HCO$_3$] mEq/l.	24	25	29	31

Fawcett and Wynn (1956) have found a much narrower range of values for these electrolytes in normal men and women in the age-range 20–35. There were small but statistically significant differences in Na, CL and CO$_2$ between men and women, but not in K. Repeated values in one individual were very constant.

words, both fluids are very nearly neutral. For practical purposes, equality of total cation and anion concentration can be assumed, so that if we know the total base concentration, the total electrolyte concentration will be double this, assuming that the mEq/l. terminology is used. This is particularly helpful in considering E.C.F, in

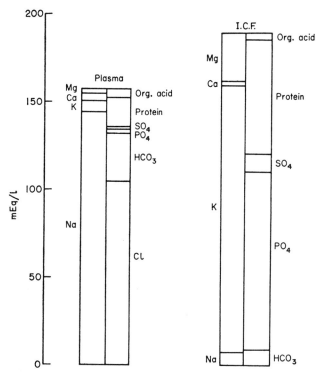

FIG. I.2. Balance of the main cations and anions in plasma and intracellular fluid. (See pp. 10–13.)

which Na makes up over 90 per cent of the total base, and in which the main anions (Cl and HCO_3) are monovalent; in this situation, doubling the Na concentrations in mEq/l. gives a value which is within 10 per cent of the total electrolyte osmolality in mM/l.

(ii) The heights of the columns representing plasma and I.C.F. are of the same order, between 150 and 200 mEq/l. This implies that there is no gross difference in electrolyte concentration between the two fluids, and such difference as there is exaggerated in the diagram, for the following reason. The chief electrolytes of plasma are monovalent, so that the number of electrical charges is the same as the number of separate particles. Inside the cells, however, the important anions are polyvalent, so that the number of particles will be appreciably less than the number of electrical charges, which is what the diagram directly represents. Similarly on the cation side, the divalent ion Mg has an osmolality which is only half its neutralizing effect as represented in the diagram. If the electrolyte concentrations presented in the diagram were converted into osmolalities, the electrolyte osmolality of plasma would be 285 mM/l. that of, I.C.F. 270 mM/l. There are, however, so many uncertainties in the determination of intracellular electrolytes, and in deciding the valence of intracellular protein and phosphate, that these figures can only be interpreted very widely as excluding a gross difference in osmolality across the cell wall. This problem is further considered in the next section, on the role of electrolytes in the body.

Turning to the differences, we would note:

(i) The preponderance of Na among the cations of E.C.F. and of K and to a less extent Mg in I.C.F. Comparative biochemistry suggests that the salinity of E.C.F. is a vestige of the marine environment in which cellular life developed (Macallum, 1926); but this may be something of a coincidence rather than a chemical necessity, for sodium can be replaced by organic bases such as choline, and yeast has been grown in a sodium-free medium. On the other hand, all cells which have been studied are rich in potassium, and there is increasing evidence that K concentration influences enzyme activity.

(ii) Among the anions, Cl and HCO_3 preponderate in E.C.F., while phosphate accounts for more than half of the anionic valences inside cells. In I.C.F., the base which is neutralized by protein is a much greater proportion of the total base than in plasma, with its comparatively low protein content; in interstitial fluid, with its low protein content, the base neutralized by protein is negligible, so that the concentration of [Na] is somewhat less than in plasma, and that of [Cl] and [HCO_3] greater. In nervous tissue, appreciable amounts of cation are associated with acidic phospholipides (Folch-Pi et al, 1957).

(iii) The [K] in E.C.F. and the [Na] in I.C.F. form a very small part of the total cation, and so make but a trivial contribution to osmolality and electroneutrality in these fluids. Nevertheless, changes in [K] of E.C.F. have been recognized as critical in the function of muscle since the work of Ringer (1883); and there is some evidence that the ill-effects of K depletion may be partly related to increase in intracellular Na (Cannon et al, 1953). Similarly the small concentrations of

TABLE 1.3

The amounts of water, Na, K, and Cl in (a) the subdivisions of E.C.F. and (b) in E.C.F., I.C.F. and total body-water. Based on figures compiled by Edelman and Leibman (1959)

	H_2O (ml/kg of body-wt.)	Na (mEq/kg of body-wt.)	K (mEq/kg of body-wt.)	Cl (mEq/kg of body-wt.)
Plasma	40	6.5	0.2	4.5
Interstitial-lymph	130	16.8	0.5	12.3
Dense connective tissue and cartilage	40	6.8	0.2	5.6
Bone	40	25	4.1	5.0
Transcellular	20	1.5	0.5	1.5
Total in E.C.F.	270	56.6	5.5	28.9
Total in I.C.F.	330	1.4	48.3	4.1
Total body-content	600	58	53.8	33.0

Ca and Mg in E.C.F. can determine 'trace effects' which are presumably unrelated to the 'bulk effects' on osmolality and electroneutrality which we have been considering.

By way of a quantitative summary of the information on distribution and electrolyte content of body-fluid, Table 1.3 sets out figures collated by Edelman and Leibman (1959). This knowledge has been chiefly built up from the results of 'space-determinations', nowadays largely carried out with isotopes. The picture is no doubt correct in its main outlines, and for normal man; but these techniques have some limitations as well as advantages. Their application in states of disease has been critically reviewed by Munro (1959) and Threefoot (1962).

At the end of this brief description of the amount, distribution and electrolyte structure of body-fluid, it may be well to attempt an outline of the general functions of electrolytes, before considering water and the individual ions in more detail.

Biological Role of Electrolytes

(1) MAINTENANCE OF ELECTRONEUTRALITY

Electrolytes are by definition ionized particles which carry a positive or negative charge and so migrate to the cathode or anode when placed in an electrical field. We have seen that in the large collections of body-fluid positively and negatively charged particles are present in such numbers that their charges are effectively neutralized. The general state of electroneutrality in body-fluid does not of course preclude local potential differences, such as exist across cell walls; between the lumen and exterior of the renal tubule; and episodically in excitable tissues such as muscle and nerve. The amount of electrolyte involved in the flux associated with nerve and muscle activity is very small in relation to the total of body-electrolyte. In this particular context, we are dealing with 'trace effects' rather than with 'bulk effects'.

(2) OSMOTIC DETERMINATION OF FLUID DISTRIBUTION

Extensive experience has shown that in health both the total electrolyte concentration and the volume of E.C.F. are maintained within quite narrow limits. If a large amount of sodium chloride is given, the electrolyte concentration rises very little, but the volume of E.C.F. increases, initially at the expense of I.C.F., though thirst soon compels an increased intake of water. Conversely, when the body is depleted of salt, the E.C.F. volume shrinks, though initially electrolyte concentration in E.C.F. is well maintained. These findings are most simply explained on the hypothesis that the amount of water in the different phases of body-fluid is determined by the number of small particles exerting an osmotic attraction to that phase (more strictly, by the lowering of aqueous vapour pressure by the presence of solute particles). The evidence of similar effects from primary changes in intracellular electrolyte is incomplete, and it is more difficult to come by, because of the difficulty of measuring I.C.F. volume with adequate precision. Indirect appraisal of the determinants of the osmolality of body-fluid can however be made either by balance techniques (the classical method) or by isotope dilution; and the results of these independent methods are in agreement. Wynn and Houghton (1957) showed that to account for changes in serum osmolality (derived from total cation concentration) it was necessary to consider not only sodium and water, but also potassium balance. Edelman et al (1958) confirmed the expected close relation between serum [Na] and serum osmolality; and showed that both these quantities were highly correlated with the expression $(Na_E + K_E)/T.B.W.$, in which Na_E and K_E are exchangeable sodium and potassium, and T.B.W. is total body-water. Moreover, serial changes in serum [Na] were highly correlated with changes in $(Na_E + K_E)/T.B.W.$, but not with changes in Na_E considered alone, or along with T.B.W., but without K_E. It can be inferred from these studies that intracellular K is osmotically active in the same sense as extracellular Na. The preponderant effect of electrolytes in deciding the amount of water in the body has been further shown by the finding of a correlation co-efficient of 0.991 between the sum of exchangeable Na and K, and the total body-water (Boling and Lipkind, 1963).

The precedence of osmolality over volume can be illustrated from the observations that a 1 per cent change in osmolality produces A.D.H. secretion (Verney, 1948), and a 1–2 per cent change initiates drinking (Wolf, 1958); whereas variations of the order of 6 per cent of the E.C.F. are tolerated without change in sodium excretion (Black, 1953), and a 10 per cent rise in body-sodium is needed to initiate secretion by the nasal salt-gland in sea-gulls (McFarland, 1964).

It is important to remember that the essential measure of osmotic effect is the number of particles present in unit volume, and not their total mass; for this explains the great importance of electrolytes in determining osmotic equilibrium in the body. Comparing protein with sodium in plasma, there is about twenty times as much protein by weight; but because of the high molecular weight of protein, and the small mass of the sodium ion, the protein osmolality is less than

2 mM/l., while that of sodium is about 140 mM/l.; moreover, the anions neutralizing sodium have a similar osmolality, so that electrolytes contribute almost all of the osmolality of plasma, which is around 300 mM/l. Small-molecule non-electrolytes, such as urea and glucose, are present in comparatively low concentration in plasma; urea contributes 5 mM/l., and glucose about the same amount. When the blood urea and blood-sugar are raised in disease, thèy then make a larger contribution to plasma osmolality. Urea cannot cause shifts of water within the body, because it is increased to about the same extent in all phases of body-fluid.* In diabetic coma, glucose may increase sufficiently to exert an osmotic effect, since it does not readily pass the cell membrane, and so may draw some water out of cells. Hyperglycaemia and hypernatraemia are often combined in such patients; but in some patients hyperglycaemia can cause significant hyperosmolality in the absence of hypernatraemia (Danowski and Nabarro, 1965). When non-electrolytes, such as mannitol or urea, become concentrated in the process of urine formation, they can exert significant osmotic action. Protein osmotic pressure also becomes significant across membranes which are permeable to water and small electrolytes, but not to protein, such as the capillary wall, including that of the glomerular loops. Nevertheless these effects of non-electrolyte osmotic action in special strategic situations should not obscure the overwhelming quantitative preponderance of electrolytes in determining osmotic balance in the body. This osmotic function of electrolytes is of great importance in health and disease, and many of the effects of excess and depletion of electrolytes, especially of sodium, can be explained in terms of osmolality. While the classical studies on sodium metabolism, such as that of McCance

---

* This statement needs qualification, in relation to brain-fluid and C.S.F. On the one hand, hypertonic urea solutions are effective in diminishing cerebral oedema (Stubbs and Pennybacker, 1960); conversely, where urea is very rapidly removed from the body, there is a lag in the clearance of urea from nervous tissue, and this is associated with confusional states and changes in the electroencephalogram (Kennedy et al, 1963). So far as we know, this state of relative impermeability to urea is limited to the nervous system, and perhaps does not involve even the whole of that, in view of the well-known observation of Verney (1957) that intra-carotid injection of urea is not an effective stimulus to the release of A.D.H.

(1936), emphasized the osmotic role of electrolytes, recent interest in potassium metabolism has brought into prominence another facet of electrolyte function, now to be considered.

(3) RELATION OF ELECTROLYTES TO ENERGY METABOLISM

In spite of the complex composition of protoplasm, and its variability in different forms of life, it can be argued that the important sources of biochemical energy are comparatively few, and that they are astonishingly similar in all forms of life (Krebs, 1954). The production of energy by anaerobic glycolysis, and by aerobic glycolysis in the citric acid cycle; and the storage of energy in available form in high-energy phosphate bonds, have a very wide biological distribution; and it is interesting to find that the concentration of electrolytes, notably K and Mg, in the medium has been shown to be critical to the activity of some of the enzymes essential to these processes. A useful list of enzymes affected by electrolyte concentration is given on p. 422 of Dixon and Webb (1964). These effects of electrolyte concentration on energy metabolism are most precisely demonstrable in studies done *in vitro*, but they can be illustrated by effects discernible in the whole organism subjected to electrolyte depletion. For example, Gardner *et al* (1950) showed that K depletion impairs the utilization of carbohydrate, and Cannon *et al* (1952) found that protein synthesis is diminished in K depletion. Such clinical phenomena as the insulin-resistant diabetes of Cushing's syndrome, and the wasting of ulcerative colitis or steatorrhoea, may at times be based in part on the potassium depletion which is known to occur in these diseases; but work on the metabolic, as opposed to the osmotic, effects of electrolyte imbalance is comparatively recent.

Although electrolytes have their part to play in maintaining the right conditions for optimum biochemical activity, they may themselves be influenced by primary impairment of energy metabolism. The very existence of a $15:1$ ratio of [Na], and a $1:20$ ratio of [K], across the wall of most cells implies an active, i.e. an energy-requiring, process both to create and to maintain it. Indeed, it can be shown that the oxygen consumption of some tissues, such as the bladder-wall and the kidney, can largely be accounted for in terms of Na-transport. The stimulation of Na-transport by aldosterone has been linked with increased synthesis of the enzymes concerned in energy-production (Edelman *et al*, 1964). In a number of disease states, in which there has been no obvious distortion of electrolyte intake or output, increase in the K concentration of serum, and fall in [Na] have been observed; this phenomenon has been particularly studied by Moore *et al* (1954), who have shown that it can occur independently of corresponding alterations in the total body content of K and Na, as measured by isotope distribution. In ischaemic muscle, the cells lose potassium and gain sodium, and it seems likely that this partial blunting of the normally sharp distinction between the electrolyte structure of E.C.F. and I.C.F. may have its basis in a partial breakdown of energy metabolism.

The general functions of electrolytes can fairly well be grouped under the headings of electroneutrality, osmolality and the provision of an apt intracellular milieu for enzyme action. However, there are in addition many special functions of individual electrolytes, such as excitation of nerve, to which we have already referred; participation of Ca in blood-clotting, in irritability of contractile tissue and in bone formation; and so on. For descriptive purposes, it is convenient to consider water and electrolytes seriatim; but it can scarcely be emphasized too much that disturbances in body-fluid are usually multiple. Our analysis of 'pure' disturbances of water and individual electrolytes will owe much to experimental work; but we shall also give examples of the inter-relations between the various 'pure' distortions, many of which have first been observed clinically. This arrangement should constitute a logical approach to the practical objective of electrolyte studies, which is the treatment of relevant clinical changes in the amount and composition of body-fluid.

CHAPTER II

WATER

The amount of water in the body, and the general features of its distribution, have already been discussed. In health, water balance is broadly preserved, although the actual output of water on a constant intake varies from day to day, in accord with similar variations in electrolyte output; this is one of several indications that the osmolality of body-fluids is conserved within narrower limits than their volume. Water *intake* comprises the water in beverages and in 'dry' foods, and the water derived from oxidation of the food; water *output* comprises the water of urine and faeces, the water expended in saturating respired air, and the water lost through the skin either insensibly or visibly. These variables differ considerably in their relative quantitative importance. The water derived from solid food (intrinsic moisture + water of oxidation) is close to 500 ml on all ordinary diets; whereas the daily intake of water as beverages may range from 500 ml to several litres, either voluntarily or in compensation for forced losses of water. Variation in the output of water by skin and lungs may be very great from one climate to another, or in patients with pyrexia; but these variations are a charge on water balance, and not a means of regulation, which on the output side is accomplished by change in urinary excretion of water. The preservation of water-balance in the face of changes in water intake and output depends mainly on two mechanisms—change in intake of beverages in response to thirst, and change in renal water output in response to the antidiuretic hormone of the posterior pituitary gland.

Thirst

We have all experienced the discomfort of thirst, and the

compensating pleasure of satisfying it. As soon as we dip below the surface of this common experience, and try to analyse it in terms of physiological stimulus and mechanism, we are in difficulties. The stimulus to thirst cannot be simply a reduction in the absolute amount of water in the body, for thirst can be regularly induced by infusion of hypertonic saline or more simply by eating salty food. We have therefore to seek a change common to deprivation of water and the addition of solute to the body; for in addition to common salt, other substances such as sorbitol, sodium sulphate and acetate have been shown to induce thirst. The obvious change of this nature is increased osmolality either of body-fluid as a whole, or of some compartment of body-fluid. It is noteworthy that sodium salts, which effectively remain in the E.C.F., are more potent in producing thirst than are equivalent amounts of urea, which penetrates cells readily. This suggests that the effective stimulus to thirst may not be a change in osmotic pressure *per se*, but some function of water loss either from the intracellular compartment as a whole, or from some specialized group of cells in an 'osmo-receptor' the same as or akin to that postulated for initiating A.D.H. secretion. Detailed evidence for cellular dehydration as a cause of thirst has been presented by Wolf (1958).

There are, however, situations both clinical and physiological, in which factors other than cellular dehydration seem to influence the intensity of thirst. It has often been stated that patients with sodium depletion do not experience thirst, because their main loss of fluid is from the extracellular compartment; but some patients seem ignorant of this, and obstinately complain of thirst when their plasma sodium is below normal limits. It is, of course, difficult for untrained observers to distinguish between ordinary thirst and the unpleasant metallic taste observed by McCance (1936) in sodium depletion; and there is evidence, reviewed by Strauss (1957) that 'pure E.C.F. volume deficiency' can be an effective thirst stimulus. Again, many accounts of clinical potassium depletion describe thirst, which can be explained in terms of diminished I.C.F. secondary to shortage of K, or as a consequence of the polyuria of potassium depletion. There is, however, a suggestion that potassium deficiency may directly stimulate the thirst centre (Fourman and Leeson, 1959).

There is also evidence from animal experiment that local factors, such as dryness of the mouth, diminished salivary flow, and gastric distension can influence thirst as judged by voluntary water consumption. In some species, such as man and the rat, voluntary water drinking falls short of the amount needed to repair an induced water deficit, suggesting that local factors can inhibit thirst before cellular rehydration is completed. A hypothalamic 'thirst centre', located between the *columna fornicis descendens* and the *tractus Vicq d'Azyr*, has been demonstrated in the goat by Andersson and McCann (1955). The existence of a similar centre in man is suggested by the record, quoted by Fourman and Leeson (1959), of a woman who lost her thirst immediately on drainage of a cyst which was pressing on the hypothalamus.

Urinary concentration and dilution

The thirst mechanism is activated by increase in the osmolality of body-fluid, and lapses when this falls, so that in effect it is a regulating mechanism only when body-fluid osmolality is normal or raised. In this, it is comparable to the operation of urinary concentration, which discharges from the body relatively more solute than water, a process which corrects hyperosmolality. But unlike the thirst mechanism, regulation by the kidneys is operative over the whole range of body-fluid osmolality, for the formation of urine of different degrees of hypo-osmolality is a homeostatic operation, dependent on the re-absorption of solute in the distal tubule. Cessation of thirst is an 'all-or-none' phenomenon, whereas urinary dilution is a graded process.

It is important, however, to differentiate between two general mechanisms whereby urine flow can be increased—*osmotic* diuresis and *water* diuresis. In osmotic diuresis, the primary event is an increase in the output of solute, which then determines an increase in the output of water, the concentrating capacity of the kidney being limited. As urine flow increases, the output of water goes up not only absolutely but also relatively to the amount of solute, so the urine becomes more dilute; its osmolality tends to fall towards that of plasma, or even a little lower. In the total process, however, solute is disposed of from the body rather than water; so that osmotic diuresis has to be regarded as an obligatory loss of water from the body, and not as a means of regulating the water household. Osmotic diuresis is well exemplified by the polyuria of diabetes mellitus, in which glucose is the loading solute. Throughout water diuresis, on the other hand, the osmolality of the urine formed is below that of plasma, and at high flow-rates it is little greater than that of tap-water. There is obviously here a mechanism for the removal from the body of water in great excess over solute; and this is a true part of water regulation. Water diuresis will increase the osmolality of body-fluid by increasing the residual solute/water ratio in the body; it is thus the converse mechanism to thirst, whose satisfaction demands and accomplishes the osmotic dilution of body fluid.

Osmotic diuresis is a mechanism whereby substantial amounts of sodium and potassium can be lost from the body; the consequent depletions are considered in later chapters. Here we have to consider water diuresis, which is relevant first as a part of the homeostasis of water; then as a cause of water depletion; and finally as a response to water excess.

The mechanism regulating urine osmolality has been reviewed elsewhere (Black, 1965, 1967). In outline, the hairpin arrangement of tubular and vascular loops in the medulla of the kidney constitutes a counter-current system (Wirz et al, 1951) which promotes a build-up of solute, based either on active sodium transport in the thick portion of the ascending limb of Henle's loop (Gottschalk, 1964), or on the hydrostatic pressure-difference between arterial and venous limbs of the vasa recta (Lever, 1965). Medullary osmolality during antidiuresis is equivalent to the osmolality of collecting-duct urine, and may thus exceed 1000 mOsm/L, in contrast to plasma osmolality of about 300 mOsm/L. In water diuresis medullary osmolality remains higher than that of plasma, even if only slightly; so that the urine formed is now much more dilute than the tissue through which it flows. Ability to form a concentrated urine would seem to depend in part on ability to establish medullary hyperosmolality; but formation of a dilute urine is not dependent on a comparable 'dilution' of medullary solute, but on the generation of solute-free water by active solute reabsorption, without accompanying water, in the distal tubule.

A central role in the response to increase in the osmolality of body-fluid is filled by antidiuretic hormone (Verney, 1957). When the effective osmolality of the blood perfusing the internal carotid artery is increased, this stimulates the formation of A.D.H. in the 'osmo-receptors' in the supra-optic and para-ventricular nuclei of the hypo-thalamus, and also the release of A.D.H. from the posterior pituitary. There are significant extrarenal actions of A.D.H. e.g. an increase in water absorption from the gut (Wakim, 1967); but its main effect is on the kidney, promoting the formation of urine of small volume

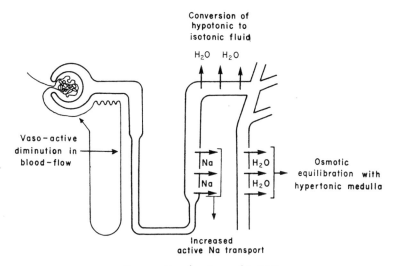

Conversion of
hypotonic to
isotonic fluid

H_2O H_2O

Vaso-active
diminution in
blood-flow

Na H_2O
Na H_2O

Osmotic
equilibration with
hypertonic medulla

Increased
active Na transport

FIG. 2.1. Renal actions of A.D.H.

and high osmolality. As indicated in Fig. 2.1, A.D.H. may increase the osmolality of the urine by several different mechanisms—the high osmolality in the medullary tissue is enhanced both by greater Na reabsorption (which adds to the trapped medullary solute) and by diminished blood-flow (which restricts 'wash-out' of solute); and the nascent urine in the collecting ducts is put into free communica-tion with its hypertonic environment, so that water reabsorption is increased in the distal nephron. In general terms, the whole mechan-ism constitutes a feed-back sequence, in which increased osmolality of plasma leads to increased concentration of the urine, which will tend to lower plasma osmolality. Acute increments of the order of

C

2 per cent in the osmolality of internal-carotid plasma are adequate to induce A.D.H. secretion; but maintained change in plasma osmolality may be associated with an altered 'set' of the osmoreceptors, since a sustained fall in plasma sodium does not inhibit A.D.H. production, and conversely a sustained rise in plasma sodium does not prevent a diuresis in response to acute water ingestion.

While the effect of increased osmolality as a stimulus to A.D.H. production is fully established, other effective stimuli are now recognized (Wakim, 1967). These include pain, apprehension, and exercise; many commonly used drugs, including morphine, barbiturates, nicotine, adrenaline, histamine, cholinergic agents, and ether; and decrease in blood-volume or in E.C.F.-volume. Conversely, A.D.H. secretion is inhibited by osmotic dilution of body-fluid; by the ingestion of alcohol; and by distension of the left atrium or central venous reservoirs.

When the water content of the body is reduced without change in the solute content, the osmolality of body-fluid increases, and stimulates the A.D.H. mechanism. The output of water in the urine is reduced, and the concentration of solutes in the urine rises correspondingly. The total excretion of electrolytes is not increased when A.D.H. action is induced by water deprivation. When A.D.H. is administered and also a large water-load, sodium excretion is somewhat increased; but this probably represents a response to increased volume of E.C.F., rather than a 'natriuretic' action of A.D.H. itself (Wrong, 1959).

The mechanisms of thirst and A.D.H. activity have several common features, which help to define their place in homeostasis. They are both readily activated by quite small changes in the osmolality of body-fluid, provided these are acutely induced; in such circumstances, the response is rapid. On the other hand, the response of both mechanisms to changes in volume of body-fluid, without change in osmolality, is comparatively insensitive and sluggish. Again, both mechanisms are activated by water deficit, and together they constitute an effective defence against it by increasing intake and lowering output; but the defence against a water-load is by inhibition of thirst and of A.D.H. release, and this defence is notably less efficient, in that 'absence of thirst' does not necessarily prevent drinking; ar 1

A.D.H. release can continue, under the influence of pain, emotion, and drugs, even when its inhibition would be called for by a positive water balance. In other words, the natural stress of water deprivation is well guarded against, whereas our defence is rather poorer against water-loading, which is only likely to occur artificially, but may then be of critical importance.

Since both mechanisms are sensitive to changes in osmolality and comparatively indifferent to volume changes, their essential role in homeostasis is to maintain osmotic constancy. It follows from this that primary changes in the solute content of the body will tend to induce equivalent changes in water content. Examples of such behaviour are given by Gamble (1951) in his monograph on the companionship of water and electrolytes in the organization of body-fluids. Increased intake of solutes induces thirst, and increased excretion of solutes carries out water in an osmotic diuresis. It must however, be recognized that companionship of water and electrolytes presupposes integrity of the mechanisms which subserve osmotic constancy; in a number of situations these fail, and we can then have gross deviations from normal osmolality. The clinical syndromes of water depletion (hyper-osmolality) and water intoxication (hypo-osmolality) will be discussed in this chapter; their occurrence depends on either breakdown or overloading of one or both of the thirst and A.D.H. mechanisms.* Syndromes which depend primarily on solute changes will be discussed in later chapters.

Polyuria

A patient with a defect of urinary concentration, but with free access to water, generally drinks enough to avoid any great measure of water depletion, so that the clinical presentation is polyuria, which

* Apart from the major mechanisms (thirst and A.D.H.) there are certainly other factors influencing the renal reabsorption of water. Many of them act primarily on electrolytes, the effect on water being secondary. However, Lindeman et al (1961) have shown increased water output, not accounted for by change in electrolyte output, under the influence of cortisone (but not of progesterone, oestrogen, or aldosterone). Conversely, after allowing for its effect on electrolyte excretion, chlorothiazide has been shown to diminish the free-water clearance (Crawford et al, 1960).

may be great enough to constitute a problem in its own right. The consequent thirst, together with the polyuria, thus constitutes the syndrome of diabetes insipidus recently reviewed by Coggins and Leaf (1967). This can arise from extrarenal and from renal causes.

Diabetes insipidus of extrarenal origin implies a lack of circulating A.D.H., and is characterized by a definite response to administered A.D.H. This may not be maximal, indeed is unlikely to be so in established diabetes insipidus, for even normal people show a transient defect in urinary concentration after polyuria has been maintained for a time by water-drinking (de Wardener and Herxheimer, 1957). Failure to concentrate the urine fully, when A.D.H. is supplied, must indicate a degree of renal defect, superimposed on the primary extrarenal causes of the polyuria; the renal abnormality may well be a lowering of medullary osmolality, such as has been shown in rats undergoing sustained forced water-diuresis (Andriole and Epstein, 1965). The two commonest extrarenal causes of the diabetes insipidus syndrome are 'true diabetes insipidus' (in the narrow sense), and compulsive water-drinking. 'True diabetes insipidus' can be defined as impaired ability to form A.D.H., or to release it, and is due to damage to the hypothalamus or neurohypophysis, such as may happen transiently after head-injury, or progressively in association with a variety of hypothalamic disorders, including basal meningitis, encephalitis, neoplasms and tuberculomata, and essential xanthomatosis (Brain, 1962). These conditions are listed, since 'true diabetes insipidus' can most confidently be diagnosed by the positive demonstration of one of these associated conditions, rather than from any of the differential tests so far available. Evidence of visual defect, or of associated hypothalamic disturbance of sleep or appetite, should be sought.

The other main extrarenal cause of the diabetes insipidus syndrome is variously known as functional or hysterical polydipsia, or compulsive water-drinking (Barlow and de Wardener, 1959). In this condition, the polyuria is more variable in degree than it is in structural diabetes insipidus; there is no evidence of structural neurological disorder, but rather of a disturbed personality; and the syndrome favours middle-aged women (possibly because disturbed men addict themselves to stronger waters).

The patient with true diabetes insipidus tends to be in marginal water depletion, the compulsive water-drinker in marginal over-hydration, and this is reflected in a raised serum-sodium in the former, and a lowered serum-sodium in the latter group. The administration of A.D.H. tends to relieve the thirst and polyuria rather dramatically in the patient with the true diabetes insipidus; whereas the other group may go on drinking, even when their urine has been made more concentrated, so that they risk water intoxication. Stimulation of the hypothalamus by nicotine or infusion of hypertonic saline should theoretically produce a concentrated urine in the compulsive water-drinker, and not in the patient who cannot form A.D.H.; but these tests have proved inferior to the natural stimulus of water-deprivation, which must however be carried out under close observation, to ensure that the compulsive water-drinker is not evading the restriction, and that the patient with true diabetes insipidus is not becoming grossly dehydrated. In more concrete terms, a patient who during water-deprivation loses 5 per cent of body-weight, and yet fails to produce a urine of osmolality higher than that of plasma, is not likely to be a compulsive water-drinker, but rather to have diabetus insipidus, which may however be 'nephrogenic' rather than 'primary'. It should be stressed again, however, that while in terms of tests there is a clear-cut statistical difference between the two major types of extrarenal 'diabetes insipidus', the problem of diagnosis in the individual patient can present real difficulty, calling for close analysis of all features of the illness, rather than any single test.

Nephrogenic diabetes insipidus. If the giving of long-acting A.D.H. (e.g. pitressin tannate in oil) fails to induce a concentrated urine, an inadequate renal response has been demonstrated. Rarely this is due to a specific inherited tubular defect, affecting mainly males, but not confined to them (Orloff and Burg, 1963). Apart from this clear-cut abnormality, impaired urinary concentration has been observed in many forms of renal disease, and is certainly not limited to conditions, such as the Fanconi syndrome or pyelonephritis, in which the tubules might be considered to be peculiarly or predominantly involved. Impaired urinary concentration is of course a feature of general renal failure, the mechanism of polyuria being largely an osmotic diuresis, each surviving nephron being called on to excrete a greater share of the total solute-load (Platt, 1952). In the absence of renal failure, defective concentrating power could be due to lack of response of the distal nephron to A.D.H., or to impairment of the counter-current mechanism which induces medullary hyperosmolality under conditions of fluid-deprivation (Black, 1965).

Water Depletion

The term 'dehydration'—which should mean a complete absence of water—has been used loosely in the past to describe at least two syndromes which we now believe to be distinct—water depletion and sodium depletion. I have argued elsewhere (Black, 1953) that the signs by which clinical dehydration is commonly assessed are more marked in sodium depletion than in water depletion of comparable degree; but some of them may be found in severe water depletion. In any case, the term 'dehydration' obscures the distinction between water and sodium depletion, and confusion here may lead to faulty treatment; so the term is now better avoided, or used as a purely descriptive term like 'wasting', which carries no precise implication as to cause or mechanism.

The contrasting effects of sodium and water depletion were observed in animals by Kerpel-Fronius (1935). During the 1939–45 war, the predicament of castaways on rafts and in the desert stimulated several experimental studies of the effects of water depletion in man.* The clinical lessons to be drawn from this work were described in detail by Marriott (1947), and his account has widely influenced the practical management of body-fluid depletion.

The experimental studies of water depletion in animals and men were naturally concerned with the pure syndrome induced by deprivation of water intake while loss of water continued through skin, lungs and kidneys. Under these conditions, loss of water is quickly diminished by a fall in urine output. The volume of urine actually formed during established water depletion depends on the amount of osmotically active solutes derived from the diet. Protein foods are degraded to urea and fixed acids, which require renal

* Nadal, Pedersen and Maddock (1941); Black, McCance and Young (1944); Winkler, Danowski, Elkinton and Peters (1944); Gamble (1946–47).

excretion; whereas fat and carbohydrate yield mainly water and carbon dioxide. On any normal diet, water deprivation quickly induces a situation in which the water available for urine formation is inadequate to excrete a normal solute load, even at maximal urine

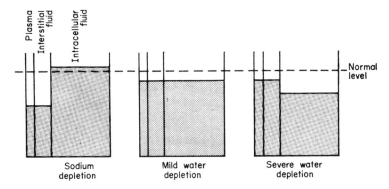

FIG. 2.2. Effect of sodium depletion, and of mild and severe water depletion, on the partition of fluid between E.C.F. and I.C.F. The partial preservation of E.C.F. at the expense of I.C.F. in severe water depletion is probably related to secondary aldosteronism. (See pp. 29, 49). Professor J. N. Hunt has drawn my attention to a difficulty in this Figure. Since there is no obvious reason why sodium–depletion should be attended by a deficiency of plasma protein (on which plasma volume depends), it might be expected that plasma volume would not be reduced to the same extent as E.C.F. volume. This is indeed the situation depicted by Marriott (1947) in a comparable diagram. However, Elkinton et al (1946) found that plasma volume was more greatly reduced than was E.C.F. volume, and indeed observed 'loss of circulating protein and of albumin in particular'. At the risk of over-simplification, I have kept the diagram in the same form as in previous editions, in the absence of any extensive figures on which a decision between these opposite views could be based.

concentration. Of necessity, the osmotic pressure of body-fluids increases while their volume diminishes; the increase of osmolality and the diminution in volume are at first spread evenly over the sub-divisions of body-fluid. Later on, however, the diminished volume of body-fluid stimulates the secretion of aldosterone (Bartter, 1958), and Na is thus conserved, so that the loss of fluid falls predominantly on I.C.F., and not on the E.C.F., which includes plasma-volume; the relative preservation of plasma-volume may have some survival value. In sodium depletion, on the other hand, the loss of fluid is extracellular, and intracellular fluid may be normal or even increased—while the osmolality of body-fluid is diminished. The contrasting effects on fluid-volume and distribution of a depletion of water and a depletion of extra-cellular electrolyte (sodium and accompanying anion) are summarized in Fig. 2.2.

The clinical syndrome of water depletion is wider than the experimental one, for it must be expanded to include not only absolute and pure water deficiency, but also relative water deficiency—a state in which the water content of the body may be normal or even increased, but the electrolyte content of the body is increased to a still greater degree. The factor common to these states is increased osmolality of body-fluid. This is usually reflected, for practical purposes, in an increase in the sodium concentration of plasma, which is a reliable index of the osmolar concentration of body-fluid in most circumstances.*

Clinical water depletion is usually induced by insufficient water intake as a result of coma, lethargy, or gastro-intestinal disease such as to prevent water ingestion or absorption. Marriott stresses the importance of sheer weakness as a cause of water depletion—'extremely enfeebled patients cannot make their need for water effective'. Specific loss of the thirst sensation has been described in hypothalamic damage from hydrocephalus and other causes, in the absence of coma (Hays et al, 1963).

Most of the body's secretions are approximately isosmotic with body-fluid, so their loss does not in itself lead to water depletion as

* Normally, the contribution of non-electrolytes to the osmolality of extra-cellular fluid is negligible (Gamble, 1954); and sodium forms more than 90 per cent of the total cation. An approximation to the total osmolality of plasma can thus be reached by doubling the plasma [Na]. In uraemia and in hyperglycaemia the non-electrolyte osmolality of plasma is significantly increased, so that estimates based on plasma sodium will under-value the osmolality of plasma. In states of hyperlipaemia, e.g. the nephrotic syndrome and xanthomatous biliary cirrhosis, plasma sodium concentrations are no longer representative of E.C.F. [Na], being substantially lower as a result of dilution of the plasma with fat (Albrink et al, 1955).

we have defined it; their loss tends rather to cause deficits of sodium or potassium. Important exceptions to this are sweat, which is normally hypotonic, and urine, which may become so. Because of the hypotonicity of sweat, patients with fever are more liable to relative water depletion. Hyperpnoea also can lead to significant water loss; the loss of water is determined by the volume of respired air and the extent to which inspired air falls short of saturation with water vapour. Significant loss of water, in excess of solute, in the urine can occur in a large number of pathological states, reviewed by de Wardener (1962). Even when we have set aside those states in which polyuria is simply an appropriate response to excessive ingestion of water, and also those in which the diuresis is osmotic, and not of water, we are still left with a number of conditions, both extrarenal and renal, which can cause water depletion by the mechanism of water diuresis (see preceding section on Polyuria).

The 'water requirement' of any given patient can only be assessed in the most general terms, because extrarenal losses of water cannot be accurately estimated, and because the need for water is related to the formation of osmotically active substances in the body, either from the diet or from breakdown of body-tissue. In fever, there is both increased extrarenal loss of water and increased catabolism of body-tissue. The importance of diet is exemplified by the relative frequency of water depletion in patients given a high-protein diet by tube-feeding; water depletion has been observed in patients whose fluid intake was over 2 litres a day, but who were also receiving over 100 g of protein in their diet (Engel and Jaeger, 1954).

Clinical water depletion has sometimes been reported in association with intracranial lesions, and 'cerebral salt retention' has been invoked to explain the consequent hypernatraemia. There are indeed many possibilities of linkage between hypothalamic activity and body-fluid, reviewed by Smith (1957), Gilbert and Glaser (1961) and Cort (1963b). But hypothalamic damage can cause diabetes insipidus; while inadequate water intake is likely in comatose patients, and can cause both water depletion and sodium retention. Whether there is any direct cerebral influence on renal sodium retention seems to me to remain doubtful; but Taylor (1962) makes a case for what he terms 'encephalogenic hypernatraemia'.

The chief difficulty in detecting water depletion, apart from remembering that such a state exists, lies in the fact that those patients who develop it are often quite unable to give an account of their condition. Patients who cannot drink often cannot speak; and severe water depletion can itself lead to mental confusion. In apathetic and confused patients, we must be assured that water is not only available, but is being consumed in adequate amount: also, the amount needed may be greater than normal. Information on urinary output is often more accurately available than information on intake; and a urine volume of over a litre a day makes serious water depletion unlikely. It does not absolutely exclude it, for a failure of renal concentrating ability allows the formation of copious and dilute urine even when the body is depleted of water. The finding of a raised plasma sodium concentration is perhaps the most definite evidence of water depletion that can be obtained in a patient who cannot give a history; provided, of course, that hypertonic saline has not been given.

In patients who are conscious and rational, the diagnosis of water depletion should present no difficulty. The patient will complain most of all of a thirst which he cannot slake; and he may also tell us how the state has arisen, whether obviously because of failure to take or retain drinks, or more subtly because of polyuria. The flow of saliva is reduced, and he may find it hard to chew and swallow his food. He may also complain of weakness, apathy and difficulty in concentrating his faculties. Physical examination shows a dry tongue and mouth, and often surprisingly little else. The hypotension, collapsed veins and low tissue-turgor of sodium depletion are not to be found in pure water depletion, except in its most advanced stages; however, the circumstances which lead to water depletion may also lead to tissue wasting, and it may be impossible to distinguish (water depletion + wasting) from primary sodium depletion simply from the appearance and feel of the subcutaneous tissues. In advanced water depletion, there may be a moderate fall in cardiac output and blood-pressure, and increase in circulation time; central nervous impairment, including respiratory failure, may be present (Elkinton and Danowski, 1955).

The urine is generally small in volume, concentrated, of high specific gravity and urea and electrolyte content. In patients with renal insufficiency, however, and also in some patients with lesions of the central nervous system, the urine may contain only traces of sodium and chloride. The plasma is invariably concentrated in respect of sodium and its accompanying anions. In contrast to sodium depletion, the loss of fluid from the plasma is matched by a corresponding loss of fluid from the erythrocytes, so that the haematocrit percentage is not raised. The plasma protein concentration is raised by about the same degree as the sodium concentration. In moderate experimental water depletion in man, a 10 per cent rise in plasma sodium was observed; but much greater increases have been recorded in patients. The most significant single observation on plasma is the increase in plasma sodium or osmolality; the changes in plasma protein are difficult to interpret without knowledge of the 'normal' level for that patient.

The treatment of water depletion is simple in principle, and also in practice when the patient can take and retain water by mouth. Intake of water should be increased until thirst has disappeared, and thereafter should be kept at a level sufficient to prevent thirst; once the depletion has been corrected, fluids should no longer be forced, but maintained at a level of 1.5 to 2 litres a day in patients not in renal failure. When the kidneys are inefficient, there is some risk of an unnoticed transition from water depletion to water intoxication; so it is specially important to tail off the water-load after the initial vigorous replacement. In conscious and co-operative patients, absence of thirst is a better guide to the absence of water depletion than is the amount of urine formed, or even a water-balance chart, which can never be complete because of metabolic gains and insensible losses of water.

In patients who are unconscious and vomiting, water depletion must be corrected and water balance maintained by rectal, subcutaneous, or intravenous fluid. If this state of affairs is likely to persist for a few days only, there is no need to supply protein and electrolytes, the main need being for water and for calories. This need can usually be supplied each day by 2 litres of 5 per cent glucose, and in adults the intravenous route is the most satisfactory. A pure carbohydrate regime must of course be supplemented by B-complex vitamins parenterally. The 100 g of glucose given in this way do not supply the energy needs of the body, and some wasting will occur; but they are sufficient to prevent the ketosis and enhanced protein catabolism of total starvation (Gamble, 1946–47). In patients who have already sustained a water deficit, more fluid has to be given at first to correct this; in the absence of the thirst criterion, correction of the deficit can only be assessed by the urine volume and the plasma sodium concentration or osmolality. Patients with fever and with polyuria obviously need more fluid to prevent water depletion. In comatose patients with no vomiting, oral tube-feeding should be used; when protein is included in the diet, the water requirement is raised, and 3 litres or more may be needed. In patients maintained for more than a few days on artificial regimes, significant deficits of sodium, potassium and other electrolytes becomes possible; their prevention and management will be discussed in later chapters.

Water Intoxication

This state has already been mentioned as a possible hazard in the enthusiastic treatment of water depletion, real or imagined; and this is indeed the way in which it most often arises. Normally, water intoxication is prevented by prompt water diuresis, which can cope with any voluntary water intake which does not cause nausea; but the same circumstances of disease which lead to inadequate fluid intake may also impair the ability to shed an imposed water-load.

Experimentally, water intoxication has been induced in animals by giving very large amounts of water by stomach-tube; or in man by giving somewhat smaller relative amounts of water by mouth, but to subjects in whom water diuresis has been inhibited by A.D.H. The effects observed in man have included fatigue, mental confusion, headache and nausea leading to vomiting; in animals, convulsions, followed by coma and death, can be regularly induced. Human subjects gain weight, their faces appear puffy, and there may be slight pitting oedema of the legs (Wrong, 1956). There is a fall in the plasma concentration of electrolytes, in the haemoglobin and plasma proteins; the haematocrit percentage does not change appreciably, indicating that the part of the water-load remaining in the blood-stream is distributed evenly between erythrocytes and plasma. Comparison of the increase in body-water and the fall in extracellular total base concentration suggests that the excess water is 'distributed between the cells and E.C.F. according to the concentration of osmotically active solutes in the two fluid compartments' (Wynn, 1955). The urine, in the absence of administered A.D.H., quickly becomes dilute, and of low concentration; nevertheless, the excretion of sodium and of chloride is augmented per unit time, even though their concentration in the urine is decreased. This natriuresis probably depends on a diminution of aldosterone secretion, in response to the induced expansion of the volume of body-fluid (Wrong, 1956).

Although the possibility of water intoxication occurring clinically was stressed by Rowntree (1922), for many years only isolated case-reports appeared, and it seems possible that many instances of water intoxication were overlooked. Appreciation of the value of fluid restriction in anuria has contributed to a revived interest in water intoxication, and two well-documented series arising in surgical practice have been published (Zimmerman and Wangensteen, 1952; Wynn and Rob, 1954). It is obvious from these and other accounts that the main causes of clinical water intoxication are inadequate urine volume, and the forced administration of hypotonic fluid by abnormal routes. Inadequate urine volume is not limited to the anuria or extreme oliguria of renal tubular necrosis or urinary obstruction. It can be induced by an excess of A.D.H. released in response to pain or trauma, or more obscurely associated with cerebral lesions or bronchial neoplasm (see p. 58); very large doses even of oxytocin have been reported to cause water intoxication (Pittman, 1963). Adrenal insufficiency, both primary and secondary to Simmonds' disease, is associated with inadequate water diuresis (Oleesky and Stanbury, 1951). Water diuresis is also inadequate in sodium depletion (McCance, 1936). (Sodium depletion is doubly harmful in this context, since it not only prevents the adequate elimination of a water-load, but is in itself as it were a half-way house on the road to water intoxication, in so far as this depends on dilution of body-fluid; Wynn and Rob (1954) have invoked losses of base to explain the appearance of water intoxication in patients who have not been grossly overloaded with water.) As regards intake of water, this is unlikely to lead to water intoxication when given by mouth at the patient's own discretion, for nausea and distaste for water appear early in water intoxication; but I have seen instances in which patients have been persuaded to take by mouth more water than was good for them. More commonly, however, the rectum or a vein has been called into service to override the patient's inclinations and tolerance. A conjunction of inadequate water diuresis and artificial forcing of fluids is possible in the day or two following operation (LeQuesne and Lewis, 1953); and it is in these circumstances that acute water intoxication has most often been reported. As Wynn and Rob (1954) point out, however, reduced ability to excrete water may persist for a week or more after operation, and be associated with small electrolyte losses; in this situation, water intoxication may come on gradually. In patients with psychological disturbance, 'compulsive water drinking' may simulate diabetes insipidus, and make the patients liable to water intoxication, especially if they are given A.D.H. in the course of investigating their polyuria (Barlow and de Wardener, 1959). The pitressin test for epilepsy sometimes led to water intoxication; and even without A.D.H., water drinking has led to intoxication in two patients with schizophrenia (Langgård and Smith, 1962). Two unusual causes of water intoxication which have been reported are colonic washouts with tap-water (Hiatt, 1951; Clayton-Jones, 1953); and fresh-water drowning, in which very large amounts of water enter the circulation via the lungs, in contrast to salt-water drowning, which is associated with haemoconcentration (Donald, 1955).

The symptoms of water intoxication vary with its degree and rapidity of onset. Those patients who become intoxicated within 48 hours of operation show predominantly cerebral symptoms, with a short period of disordered behaviour followed by convulsions, which may be succeeded by fatal coma if the condition is not recognized and treated. The blood-pressure may be increased to a moderate degree, and the circulation is well maintained. The sub-cutaneous tissues are well hydrated. Unequal pupils, altered reflex activity and extensor plantar responses have been observed. In patients who develop water intoxication more gradually, the clinical picture is less definite, with lethargy and prostration, muscle weakness, sleepiness, apathy and disorientation (Wynn and Rob, 1954). Thirst is almost always absent.

The diagnosis of water intoxication is largely a matter of awareness of the circumstances in which it is likely to occur. It should be suspected when a neurological or psychological disturbance follows operation or a period of oliguria. The most consistent biochemical evidence of water intoxication is a reduced plasma sodium concentration or osmolality. While a normal plasma sodium level excludes water intoxication as a cause of symptoms, a low plasma sodium level may be related not to water intoxication, but to sodium depletion or to 'symptomless hyponatraemia' (Wynn and Rob, 1954; Wynn, 1956). Sodium depletion severe enough to lower the plasma concentration of sodium will declare itself in unequivocal dehydration; moreover, in severe water intoxication, the plasma sodium is often under 120 mEq/l. Those levels of plasma sodium are not observed either in uncomplicated sodium depletion, or in symptomless hyponatraemia. In the absence of an adequate history, as in a comatose patient, the diagnosis of water intoxication may have to be reached by way of a trial injection of 50 ml of 5 per cent saline. This procedure is safe in any patient with a low plasma sodium concentration, and it will alleviate the severe symptoms of water intoxication, while it is without effect on patients with sodium depletion or symptomless hyponatraemia.

Water intoxication can be prevented by restricting the intake of non-saline fluid to an amount not exceeding the urine volume by more than a litre. If water intoxication has been allowed to appear, the intake of non-saline fluid should be reduced to a minimum, and loss of water from the body encouraged by sweating, which may be conveniently induced by a radiant-heat cradle. Acute severe water intoxication, with convulsions or coma, should be treated with 5 per cent saline, in injections of 50–100 ml, repeated at hourly intervals until convulsions are controlled; the plasma sodium concentration should be estimated between each treatment, not in order to attain the biochemical perfection of a normal plasma sodium level, but to prevent over-dosage. When the plasma sodium level is up to 130 mEq/l., intravenous saline can be discontinued. The effectiveness of hypertonic saline indicates that the symptoms of water intoxication are related to the hypotonicity of body-fluid, and not to the increase in its amount. Isotonic saline is ineffective and possibly harmful in water intoxication.

CHAPTER III

SODIUM

Amount and Distribution

The total amount of sodium in the body can only be determined by chemical analysis of the whole body, which has rarely been carried out. An estimate of the sodium in the body can be made by determining the amount of sodium in which either the short-life isotope (^{24}Na) or the long-life isotope (^{22}Na) becomes diluted. Isotope dilution does not measure all the sodium in the body, more than a quarter of which is 'non-exchangeable' (Wilson et al, 1954); but it probably measures the sodium in the body which is metabolically quickly available, and this includes a substantial part of the sodium in bone (Edelman et al, 1954). In rats at least, the Na content of the fluid phase of bone is promptly affected by hypo- and by hyper-natraemia; but in 3–4 days the Na in the bone crystals is also involved (Forbes and McCoord, 1965). The greater part of the exchangeable sodium in the body is in the extracellular fluid; the remainder is in intracellular fluid and in bone. Estimates of the total and the exchangeable Na, and the amounts in E.C.F., I.C.F. and bone, are summarized in Table 3.1. As between men and women, there is only a small difference in exchangeable sodium, the mean being 41.7 mEq/kg for men, and 40.1 for women (Widdowson and Dickerson, 1964).

Although the direct estimates of Na in man are so few, the results in other species likewise show a very considerable excess of total over exchangeable Na. The greater part of the discrepancy is accounted for by the results of Edelman et al (1954) who showed that the total amount of sodium in bone had been grossly underestimated by previous methods, and that some 50 per cent of the large amount of sodium in bone was not exchangeable in the relevant time. Urist (1962) has pointed out that the sequestration of mineral in bone may have played a key role in the evolution of body-fluid in the marine vertebrates, allowing them to develop body-fluid with an osmolality only a quarter that of sea-water.

Survey of the literature (Threefoot, 1962) gives values for exchangeable Na ranging from 32.3–59.8 mEq/kg. This wide range

TABLE 3.1

Amount and distribution of sodium

	No. of subjects	mEq/kg Mean	Range	mEq/70 kg	Source
Total Na	2	75	—	5250	Widdowson *et al* (1951)
Exchangeable Na	25	41.9	32.3–54.1	2933	Forbes and Perley (1951)
Extracellular Na		25	—	1750	Calculated
Intracellular		3	—	210	Calculated
Bone Na	4	23	—	1610	Edelman *et al* (1954)

carries the practical implication that single estimates are of little value in clinical problems. Serial estimates in the same subject, or results in a group of similar patients, may be useful in investigation; and Wilson *et al* (1954) found reasonable concordance between the differences in successive estimates of exchangeable Na and the change expected from the Na balance in the interval. Since prolonged balance study involves cumulative errors, repeated estimates of exchangeable Na may be more valid in the long-term study of the sodium household in a given patient.

Sodium Homeostasis

Different people, and the same people from time to time, take very different amounts of salt in their diet. Not many people take less than 50 mEq of Na, or more than 300 mEq; but within this range intakes are evenly spread. Although gross salt deprivation, as on the rice diet, leads to a desire for salt, there is little evidence that the normal variation in salt intake is an important factor in regulating the sodium balance. In contrast to the urgency of thirst in water depletion, there is little or no 'craving for salt' in sodium depletion.[*] In default of such a craving, many immigrants to the tropics drift into the 'heat exhaustion' of mild Na depletion (Ladell *et al*, 1944). Likewise, the variation in Na loss in the sweat is not regulatory, but something imposed by climatic conditions; with this reservation, that salt loss in sweat is mitigated by a lowering of the Na concentration after some time (Dill, 1938). Losses of Na in the stool are small, and do not vary greatly in the absence of diarrhoea, although there is some evidence that mineralocorticoids increase the absorption of Na not only in the colon, but also in the small intestine (Goulston *et al*, 1963). The burden of compensating for variations in intake and in extrarenal loss falls on the kidneys.[†]

On a constant diet, and in the absence of visible sweating, the urinary output of sodium shows fluctuations from day to day of as much as 50 per cent of the mean output. Within the day, there is a well-marked diurnal (or 'circadian') rhythm (Mills, 1966) whose precise characters vary from subject to subject, but are very constant in the same individual; the highest rate of sodium excretion, which is usually in the forenoon, may be ten-fold the lowest rate, usually at night (Stanbury and Thomson, 1951). In spite of these striking changes in Na output over short periods, the Na content of the body over long periods is not grossly variable. Schottstaedt *et al* (1958) made the interesting observation that acute psychological disturbances tend to be associated with a loss of electrolyte and water from the body; while chronic states of depression are associated with

[*] This generalization does not apply to herbivorous species, in whom the large alkaline tide and the high K content of their diet create a need for salt. Denton (1965), from his study of sheep, believes that this need is partly satisfied by a neurally mediated salt-appetite, a concept which he expresses in this elegant sentence— 'Though the central nervous development of these creatures is probably, of necessity, limited by the basic circumstances of commitment to a life largely occupied by the munching of low-calorie food, nonetheless their higher nervous activity is clearly of great importance to detection and evasion of predators, inclusive of grazing and alarm behaviour of the herd, as well as their chemical self-regulation by selective appetite.'

[†] This statement is true of mammals; but it is interesting to note that the Humboldt penguin (and also some reptiles) has nasal mucous glands, which in response to increased salt intake can secrete fluid of [Na] up to 800 mEq/l. (Schmidt-Nielsen and Sladen, 1958).

fluid retention. However, the papers which have since appeared are rather conflicting; and the findings in depressive states were not confirmed by Coppen *et al* (1962). The normal diurnal rhythm was less marked in 36 patients with 'endogenous depression' than in 43 patients with 'personality disorders and neuroses'; sodium and chloride were more affected than potassium and water, and there was a tendency for the amplitude of diurnal variation to be less in older people (Elithorn *et al*, 1966). The general question of electrolyte changes in psychiatric disorders is reviewed by Shaw (1966); the relevance of these changes is supported by the encouraging results of lithium treatment in selected patients.

A large amount of detailed information has accumulated on the renal handling of sodium. Here we can mention only the main features of the process, those whose aberration is thought to lead to Na excess and depletion of renal origin. At normal rates of G.F.R. and normal plasma [Na], the amount of sodium filtered at the glomeruli lies between 13 and 20 mEq per minute; the amount of Na appearing in the urine is usually 20–300 μEq/min., which represents less than 2 per cent of the original filtered load. It is clear from this analysis that the tubules in respect of Na are quantitatively an organ of reabsorption; and this process is active, consuming energy and correlated with renal oxygen consumption (Thaysen *et al*, 1961). It is also apparent that quite minor variations in either the large amount of Na filtered, or the large amount of Na reabsorbed could readily account for impressive changes in the amount of Na finally excreted (Fig. 3.1). Lack of precision in our estimates both of G.F.R. and of plasma [Na] has been the basis of a controversy in which Homer Smith has championed small variations in sodium filtration as the means whereby sodium output is regulated; while others have devised experiments to indicate that variation in tubular reabsorption of Na is of physiological significance. I have reviewed the evidence in this matter at some length (Black, 1952); at present, I need only emphasize that these two mechanisms do not exclude one another, and one or other may be critical in any given situation. For example, in cardiac failure the great decrease in filtration rate is probably a major cause of Na retention and oedema, whereas in Addison's disease the loss of Na is clearly based on a failure of tubular reabsorption. It should be noted further that an analysis of urinary Na output in terms of filtration and reabsorption of Na is not necessarily complete; for Chinard and Enns (1955) have made the intriguing observation that when radioactive sodium and 'glomerular substances' such as creatinine are injected together into the renal

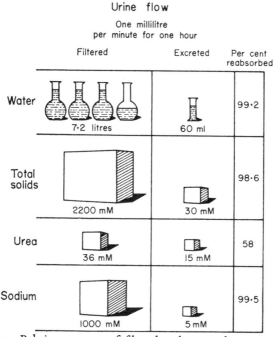

FIG. 3.1. Relative amounts of filtered and excreted water, total solids, urea and sodium.

artery, the sodium appears more quickly in the urine than the substances presumed to be filtered—suggesting that some at least of the urinary Na is contributed directly from the tubule cells.

Since urinary Na is such a small proportion of filtered Na, there must be normally a high correlation between filtered Na and reabsorbed Na; when this breaks down in disease, the situation is sometimes referred to as 'glomerulo-tubular imbalance'. It is not perhaps too obvious that this phrase is merely descriptive, and will not become explanatory until we know more of the factors which determine the more normal situation of 'glomerulo-tubular balance'.

Some information on this difficult matter is now accruing from micro-puncture work. For instance, Thurau and Schneeman (1965) showed that micro-injection of hypertonic saline into the distal tubule led to diminished filtration in the corresponding glomerulus, indicated by collapse of the proximal tubule. More recently it has been observed that increase in diameter of the proximal tubule increases Na-reabsorption (Rector et al, 1966), whereas decrease in diameter diminishes Na-reabsorption (Brunner et al, 1966). Such experiments indicate ways in which sodium-load and sodium-reabsorption could influence one another. These short-term intrarenal effects would of course be supplemented by longer-term extrarenal haemodynamic and hormonal effects. For example there is now considerable evidence, reviewed by Davis et al (1967), for a humoral natriuretic factor in saline-loaded animals, and also for a non-adrenal sodium-retaining factor in oedematous states.

The stimulus which induces the kidneys to excrete different amounts of Na has proved as debatable as the mechanism by which they effect the change. The two problems are not indeed entirely separate; for emphasis on a G.F.R. mechanism implies a change in cardiac output, or in the volume of plasma or E.C.F., as a stimulus; while emphasis on tubular reabsorption directs attention to the difficult question of what causes variation in the output of sodium-retaining hormones by the adrenal glands. The situation has been clarified to some extent by the discovery that almost all the salt-retaining activity of the adrenals is mediated by a single steroid of known chemical composition, aldosterone, which has been detected in urine, in adrenal tissue and in adrenal vein blood (Simpson, Tait and Bush, 1952), and isolated (Reichstein et al, 1963). As with most biological milestones, this important discovery concentrated on a new and profitable field of inquiry efforts which had previously been dissipated in the observation of phenomena based on so many variables as to elude reasonable interpretation. But even the right questions may not have simple answers; and there is some conflict of evidence and opinion on the nature of the stimulus to aldosterone production. Some of the discrepancies are due to the methods used; biological assays of aldosterone have gradually and irregularly been supplanted by physico-chemical methods, and estimates of excretion by that of secretion (Cope *et al*, 1962) or of plasma-level (Wolff and Torbica, 1963).

There is now considerable evidence for a number of separate stimuli and for at least two integrated mechanisms for the regulation of aldosterone activity—one mechanism having the broad characteristics of a reflex, and thus laying emphasis on nervous pathways and central representation; the other humoral, based on the renin-angiotensin system and so having its 'trigger' in the kidneys rather than in cephalad 'volume-receptors'. Unlike the glucocorticoids aldosterone is produced in the outermost layer of the adrenal cortex, the zona glomerulosa; and A.C.T.H. is not an important factor, although it may marginally enhance the production of aldosterone by increasing precursor steroids such as progesterone and corticosterone (Mulrow and Ganong, 1961). More direct stimuli to aldosterone activity include sodium restriction, potassium loading, and 'any reduction in the fullness of the blood-vessels, however produced' (Fourman, 1962). Although increase in plasma [K] and decrease in plasma [Na] have now been shown to increase the output of aldosterone in the adrenal vein (Davis *et al*, 1963), most investigation has been concentrated on volume changes, including those which occur in the passive erect posture (Brown *et al*, 1966). The general physiological aspects of volume-receptors, and their relation to baroreceptors and the hypothalamus have been reviewed by Homer Smith (1957), Wrong (1959), and Gauer and Henry (1963). In specific relation to aldosterone, a dual mechanism has been suggested by Bartter and his colleagues (1960): aldosterone secretion is stimulated by impulses arising in the junction of the carotid and thyroid arteries, and depressed by impulses arising in the atria, and transmitted in the vagus. This is certainly an arrangement capable of monitoring volume-change both in the low-pressure venous bed, and in the high-pressure arterial circulation to the brain; but the central connections remain obscure, and also the efferent mechanism to the adrenals. In one formulation, this might even be humoral, arising in the pineal (Farrell, 1958). Even these multifarious possibilities cannot be exhaustive or complete; for in the decapitated dog the response of aldosterone secretion to haemorrhagic depletion of blood-volume persists (Davis *et al*, 1961). The response was, however, abolished by nephrectomy, and at about the same time it was observed that salt deprivation led to enlargement of the renal juxtaglomerular bodies, the probable source of renin. Oligaemia and inferior vena-caval constriction both diminish renal blood-flow, and both are associated with increased aldosterone output; it is suggested that renal ischaemia stimulates the zona glomerulosa of the adrenals by means of renin, or of angiotensin. Injection of angiotensin into the adrenal artery is followed after some 3 minutes by a large increase in aldosterone secretion (Blair-West et al, 1966). The relevance of this work to sodium homeostasis has been much increased by the demonstration that in normal man sodium depletion increases the circulating renin, while sodium loading diminishes it (Brown et al, 1963).

The general effect of aldosterone on the kidney is to increase the reabsorption of Na in the distal tubule, and to increase the secretion of K and of hydrion at the same site. This at once suggests an enhancement of ion-exchange but there is some evidence that the effects on Na and on K transport are independent; for example, the retention of Na under the influence of aldosterone is transient, whereas the loss of K persists even after Na excretion has returned to normal. This phenomenon of the 'escape' of Na retention from mineralocorticoid activity had already been observed with DCA; together with the persistence of diurnal electrolyte rhythm and postural variations in Na output, it shows that aldosterone cannot be the only determinant of Na excretion. Conversely, the action of aldosterone on Na transport is not limited to the kidney; it enhances Na-reabsorption from sweat, saliva and succus entericus. So far as is known, however, the renal action is the most important, and may well account for many of the observed variations in Na excretion. There is, for example, evidence derived from the use of the steroid antagonist spironolactone that renal electrolyte excretion in normal subjects is under adrenal influence for the greater part, if not the whole, of the 24 hours (Mills et al, 1962). Since there is a delay of 30 minutes or more in any renal action of aldosterone, it cannot account for very rapid responses, such as the effects of saline infusion or venesection, which increase or diminish Na excretion within a few minutes. Also, the 'escape' phenomenon, just mentioned, limits the relevance of aldosterone to chronic Na retention.

Although aldosterone is the most important natural hormone with very great sodium-retaining action, the synthetic substance desoxy-corticosterone (DCA) is of comparable potency; and other steroids such as cortisone have some salt-retaining action, which is probably of no physiological consequence, but can become of practical importance when large doses are being given in treatment. Both cortisone and hydrocortisone have this action in high dosage, and the halogenated corticosteroids such as fludrocortisone have a pronounced salt-retaining effect; on the other hand glucocorticoids dehydrogenated at the 1 position, such as prednisone, have much less effect on Na excretion. Sodium retention can be induced by methyltestosterone (Fourman, 1952), and also by oestrogens, an effect which is responsible for pre-menstrual oedema (Thorn *et al*, 1938); salt retention sufficient to cause oedema and dyspnoea may be observed in patients with carcinomatosis on androgen or oestrogen treatment. Synthetic androgens such as norethisterone also cause Na retention; whereas progesterone, sometimes used in the palliation of 'premenstrual tension', has a natriuretic effect (Jenkins, 1961). Patients with myxoedema have Na retention, and in them thyroxin induces a natriuresis; on the other hand, excess of thyroid hormone does not affect sodium metabolism, apart from the general wasting. The anterior pituitary does not appear to affect Na metabolism directly, but indirect effects are possible either through the renotrophic action of growth-hormone, or the change in adrenal activity induced by ACTH; the small importance of the pituitary gland itself in Na metabolism is exemplified in the difference between the 'electrolytic health' of Simmonds' disease and the dehydration of Addison's disease, in which the gross Na depletion is based on lack of aldosterone, and not of the hormones directly under pituitary control. Although hyponatraemia is not uncommon in patients with hypopituitarism (Bethune and Nelson, 1965), it is related to impaired excretion of water, and not to excessive excretion of sodium. The hormones of the adrenal medulla have some action on Na excretion, largely by virtue of their vasomotor actions both general and renal; the immediate effects are largely dependent on the direction of the change in blood-pressure, but a fall in renal circulation is rather constant. It is therefore of some interest that Blake (1955) observed a constant and sustained retention of sodium which outlasted the vasomotor disturbance; this could well be due to aldosterone secreted in response to the period of renal ischaemia. Infusions of angiotension promote Na retention in normal subjects, but a natriuresis in hypertensive subjects (Brown and Peart, 1962). Laragh *et al* (1963) have now shown a striking natriuresis in patients with cirrhosis given angiotensin infusion; they suggest, moreover, that angiotensin may play a part in normal sodium homeostasis by a direct action on the renal tubules, and apart from its recognized effects on blood-pressure and aldosterone output. Slaton and Biglieri (1965) observed that in renal hypertension there was a tendency to hyponatraemia, in contrast to the high plasma [Na] found in hypertensive patients with primary aldosteronism; they suggest that in the case of renal hypertension, angiotensin may 'over-ride' the sodium-retaining action of aldosterone. Pituitary A.D.H. has no important direct action on Na excretion; when A.D.H. administration is combined with waterloading, natriuresis occurs. Insulin is not known to have any direct effect on Na metabolism; but the acidosis and hyperglycaemia of diabetic ketosis can produce severe Na depletion.

An external Na turnover of 60 to 300 mEq/day represents only 2 to 10 per cent of the exchangeable Na, and a smaller proportion of the total Na of the body. Much larger amounts of sodium, of the order of 1000 mEq, are secreted each day into the alimentary tract; but these are almost totally reabsorbed, and so do not appear in the normal Na balance. But when alimentary secretions are lost or withdrawn, their loss causes severe Na depletion. Even this large alimentary exchange of Na is much smaller than the strictly internal exchanges of Na between plasma and E.C.F., and between E.C.F. and I.C.F. These internal exchanges of Na are hard to study; but they are not without importance, e.g. the Na retention of hypoproteinaemia has as its primary cause an imbalance between plasma volume and E.C.F. volume, and the subsequent distortion of external Na and water balance is secondary. An altered equilibrium between extracellular and intracellular Na has perhaps been clearly shown only in potassium depletion; but it may also be concerned in some of the 'low-salt syndromes' not linked with K depletion.

Sodium Depletion

A rigorous definition of sodium depletion would include only those states in which the total amount of sodium in the body is reduced and this state of true sodium depletion is the main subject of the present section. For convenience, however, we include in it some account of various so-called 'low-sodium syndromes' in which the plasma [Na] is low, but the total body-sodium is not necessarily decreased. The term 'sodium depletion' should be limited to those states in which sodium has actually been lost from the body, and not stretched to include a fall in sodium concentration; this point of terminology is stressed mainly in order to discourage the belief that a low plasma sodium level is in itself an indication for giving sodium salts.

The paramount importance of sodium depletion in causing many of the symptoms and signs of clinical dehydration was first demonstrated by the *experimental studies* of Kerpel-Fronius (1935) in animals, and of McCance (1936) in man. We have already (p. 28) outlined the main features of pure water depletion; the effects of pure sodium depletion are strikingly different, forming the other extreme of a range within which fall the clinical states of body-fluid depletion. The amount of fluid held in the extracellular fluid compartment depends to a first approximation on the amount of sodium in the body; initially, McCance's subjects passed a dilute urine, so losing water in amounts comparable to the forced loss of sodium, and they maintained in this way a normal concentration of plasma sodium at the expense of E.C.F volume. With advancing sodium depletion, water loss no longer kept pace with sodium loss, and the concentration of plasma sodium fell (most patients with clinical sodium depletion are first seen at this stage). With a pure sodium depletion, not all of the water lost from the E.C.F. actually leaves the body; some of it enters the I.C.F., whose volume is increased and osmotic concentration diminished (Darrow and Yannet, 1935; Metcoff *et al*, 1957). The effects of sodium depletion are very largely those of diminished E.C.F. volume, which includes both plasma and interstitial fluid. The deficiency of plasma fluid is indicated by a rise in haematocrit and plasma-protein concentration, and by a low volume of distribution of vital red, Evans' blue, or radio-iodinated human serum albumin (RIHSA). It is reflected in poor venous filling, diminished cardiac output and a fall in systemic blood-pressure, which may be present in the recumbent subject, or may only appear on standing. (With severe clinical sodium depletion, the hypovolaemia induces tachycardia; and selective vasoconstriction diminishes the circulation through the skin and extremities, leading to cold limbs and 'dehydration fever'; and also through the kidneys, leading to oliguria and even anuria.) The diminution in interstitial fluid is indicated by a loss of tissue elasticity and 'turgor', and by low intra-ocular tension. These volume effects do not account for some of the changes observed in sodium depletion, such as muscle cramps, gastric atony with anorexia and sometimes vomiting, and in animals a lowering of the electro-convulsive threshold—these are possibly the effects of body-fluid dilution, since they are also observed in water intoxication without depletion of total body-sodium. More rapid tissue-breakdown has been observed to occur in dogs subjected to Na depletion, and this effect was seen whether the adrenals were present or not (Santos, 1959).

Clinical sodium depletion has been observed in many diseases, and a catalogue of these would make tedious and unprofitable reading. Fortunately, the mechanisms of clinical sodium loss are limited in number, and we can usefully confine our survey to those 'final common paths' to sodium depletion. A low intake of sodium does not in itself lead to significant sodium depletion, for it is quickly balanced by efficient renal conservation of sodium; but it may aggravate sodium depletion determined by other causes. The important causes of sodium depletion are abnormal losses in alimentary secretions, urine and sweat. Losses of alimentary secretions by vomiting, diarrhoea, aspiration or discharge from fistulae are the most frequent cause of severe sodium depletion, which is usually complicated by alkalosis or acidosis, depending on the higher or lower concentration of hydrion in the lost fluid. Alimentary secretions are approximately isotonic with E.C.F., and with the exception of gastric juice contain sodium in similar concentration to E.C.F.; loss of these fluids may amount to several litres a day, and the situation may be aggravated by deprivation of sodium intake*. Normal stools contain very little

* The stools in cholera may amount to 700 ml/hour, and have an electrolyte composition of [Na] 140, [K] 10, [CL] 110, and [HCO$_3$] 40 mEq/L. (Phillips, 1966).

sodium; formed stools in steatorrhoea contain some extra sodium in combination with fatty acids; but really large losses of sodium by the bowel are found only in watery diarrhoea, which can induce fatal sodium depletion in a few hours in conditions such as cholera (Watten *et al*, 1959) and the staphylococcal enteritis which may occur in association with the use of chlortetracycline and tetracycline. Mucinous discharges are rich in sodium, and sodium depletion is regularly present in patients with mucin-secreting villous tumours of the rectum and colon, some of whom are without frank watery diarrhoea (Shnitka *et al*, 1961; Wells *et al*, 1962). Sweating is a less common cause of severe sodium depletion; water is lost in excess of salt, so the most immediate effect of sweating is to cause predominantly water depletion; when this is repaired by water alone, the cumulative loss of salt becomes significant, and can lead to moderate sodium depletion, as in the heat exhaustion syndrome (Ladell *et al*, 1944). In fibrocystic disease, the [Na] in sweat is higher than normal, and patients with this disorder are prone to Na depletion and heat exhaustion (Gibson and Cooke, 1959). Exudates and transudates have the sodium concentration of E.C.F., but are not commonly lost in large enough amount to cause significant sodium depletion; an important exception is loss of ascitic fluid by paracentesis, which may cause shock from loss of sodium and of protein (Nelson *et al*, 1951).

Urinary losses of sodium are perhaps of special clinical interest, as they are more likely to go unrecognized for a time than losses of alimentary secretions; yet they can easily be documented from the volume and sodium content of the urine. Polyuria does not in itself lead to sodium depletion; patients with diabetes insipidus have a normal sodium balance, and so do many patients with moderate renal failure. Conversely, the absence of polyuria does not exclude urinary loss of sodium; patients with Addison's disease are often oliguric, though the situation here is complicated by the effect of established sodium depletion in decreasing the renal circulation. It is therefore necessary to determine the 24-hour output of sodium in the urine, rather than to attempt any inferences from urine volume alone. Excessive urinary loss of sodium may be related to lack of the aldosterone stimulus to sodium reabsorption, as in Addison's disease which is in this respect controlled by deoxycortone. A commoner cause of urinary loss of sodium is osmotic diuresis; here the loading solute may be glucose (diabetic coma) or urea (recovery from acute renal failure). Sodium depletion has been observed in the polyuric phase of acute tubular necrosis, and after relief of chronic urinary obstruction (Bricker *et al*, 1957); in these syndromes, urea diuresis and residual tubular damage may both be concerned in the loss of sodium. An interesting example of renal sodium loss has been described by Barraclough (1966) in a patient with malignant hypertension; he suggested that the saline diuresis here might be akin to the 'Druckdiurese' induced experimentally by raising the pressure at which the kidney is perfused. Another mechanism of urinary loss of sodium is in association with increased output of anions such as chloride (mercurial diuresis), keto-acids (the ketosis of diabetes and starvation) and phosphate and sulphate (increased protein catabolism). With healthy kidneys, sodium loss by this mechanism is transient, and the sodium is then 'spared' by increased renal production of ammonia; but in renal and adrenal failure, ammonia production is defective.

In chronic renal failure, the renal output of Na is related to the residual G.F.R., but does not fall in direct proportion to it (Platts, 1966). There seems to be little change in Na excretion until the impairment of renal function has progressed so far as to enforce a rise in blood-urea. At this point, the remaining nephrons are working under conditions of osmotic diuresis, in which Na excretion is increased. The consequent loss of Na is usually only moderate, but has in certain patients been great enough to justify the term 'salt-losing nephritis' (Thorn *et al*, 1964; Stanbury and Mahler, 1959; Walker *et al*, 1965). In terminal renal failure, however, the extreme loss of filtering surface may lead to enforced Na retention, which may then be a factor in promoting greater hypertension. This in turn may lead to cardiac failure, which decreases the already low G.F.R. In such patients, Na restriction, or therapeutic (dialytic) depletion, may control the hypertension more effectively than the usual hypotensive drugs. Pathological loss of salt occurs when urinary obstruction is suddenly relieved (Bricker, 1967). The extra-renal losses of salt which arise in chronic renal failure from vomiting and diarrhoea are palliated to some extent by the use of a controlled low-protein diet (Shaw *et al*, 1965).

Many of the effects of clinical sodium depletion have already been mentioned as those of experimental sodium depletion, but the effects of sodium depletion on the kidneys deserve fuller attention, in relation to the preceding paragraph on renal causes of sodium loss. With mild dietary sodium depletion, sodium practically disappears from the urine in a few days, and this process is probably mediated by increased formation of aldosterone, and does not depend on any detectable change in plasma sodium level or G.F.R. When sodium has been lost from the body in larger amount by extrarenal routes, the fall in cardiac output leads to a reduction in renal blood-flow and G.F.R.; active vasoconstriction of renal vessels lowers the renal blood-flow to a still greater extent than the mere fall in cardiac output would account for by itself. Under these conditions, the excretion of urea falls, and the blood urea level rises, it may be to several hundred mg/100 ml. This 'extrarenal uraemia' of sodium depletion may simulate primary renal failure with sodium loss. As a rule, the two conditions can be distinguished by the very low sodium output in extrarenal uraemia due to sodium depletion, in contrast to the normal or raised sodium output in sodium depletion of renal origin; but in patients with renal disease, some extrarenal uraemia may also occur, and may be detectable only by a therapeutic trial of sodium salts, which may substantially lower the blood urea level (Black and Williams, 1962). Albuminuria can occur from kidneys damaged by primary sodium depletion, but haematuria and casts point to an intrinsic renal lesion, though their absence does not exclude it. A past history of renal disease has positive value, but its absence has little negative value in this particular distinction. The error of regarding a reversible extrarenal uraemia as chronic renal failure must be avoided by close attention to the general evidence of sodium depletion, and on occasion by actual trial of sodium salts.

As might be expected the clinical picture of sodium depletion varies with the magnitude of the sodium loss, and the time over which it has developed. The mildest states of sodium depletion are seen in normal subjects who have been on the rice-diet for a few days, and have lost 100–150 mEq of sodium, and in patients exposed to tropical conditions with no special care to replace sodium losses in sweat—the 'heat exhaustion, type II' of Ladell et al, 1944. Under these conditions, there is some loss of appetite and energy, but no circulatory change, other than a diminished ability to stand quietly without fainting (DiGiovanni and Birkhead, 1964). Subjects in this state are susceptible to water-loading, and develop cramps more readily than normal subjects. Larger deficits of sodium, of the order of 300–500 mEq, are commonly found in patients with diabetic coma (Nabarro et al, 1952); at this level of sodium depletion, the deficiency of interstitial fluid and of plasma volume begins to be clinically apparent. Acute losses of fluid from the alimentary tract also produce depletion of this degree. The most severe depletion of sodium is found in patients with massive or sustained losses of fluid from the alimentary tract; such patients may retain as much as 1500 mEq of sodium before replacement is complete. They are in profound shock, and their tissues are inelastic.

The diagnosis of sodium depletion depends mainly on a knowledge of its causes and of the different clinical pictures which it may produce. Biochemical studies are of limited value in diagnosis, for the concentration of plasma sodium does not accurately reflect the state of sodium balance, since it may be affected by changes in water balance, and by shifts of sodium into or out of cells and possibly bone. A normal plasma sodium should not prevent a trial of sodium salts in a patient who is clinically dehydrated or who seems likely from his history to have lost sodium. Conversely, a low level of plasma sodium is not in itself an indication for treatment with sodium salts. These are not, of course, arguments against estimating the plasma sodium, but against placing undue emphasis on the result when it appears to contradict the clinical evidence. The chloride, bicarbonate and potassium concentration in plasma should also be estimated, as a guide to whether sodium should be given as chloride or as lactate, and whether potassium salts are also necessary. The blood urea is raised in sodium depletion great enough to interfere with renal circulation, and this may give information on the magnitude of the depletion, especially in those patients in whom clinical dehydration is difficult to assess because of wasting, or in whom concurrent congestive failure obscures the signs based on a low plasma volume. Haemoglobin, haematocrit and plasma protein estimations are difficult to assess except when they are done serially and previous 'normal' values in that patient are known. Balance studies give only retrospective information, and measurements of exchangeable sodium are likewise not immediately available. Both of these techniques have added substantially to our knowledge of Na metabolism in defined groups of patients; but their value in the management of individual patients is very limited—in the case of balance techniques by errors of collection and measurement; and in the case of E_{Na} because of the wide range of normal variation.

The treatment of sodium depletion depends on its degree. For minor depletion of sodium the addition of salt to the diet is effective both in treatment and in prevention. The salt may be added to food, taken as tablets, or dissolved in fluids; although 0.45 per cent salt in fluids tastes brackish, many patients with sodium depletion tolerate fluids with 0.9 per cent salt. When sodium depletion is of moderate degree, as in diabetic coma, and when there is some circulatory impairment and gastric atony, treatment with 0.9 per cent saline intravenously is satisfactory, since the amount needed is only 2–3 litres; this can be given by drip transfusion without overloading the circulation. When there is a complicating acidosis, part of the sodium should be given as bicarbonate or lactate; but in the absence of pre-existing acidosis, the acidifying effect of sodium chloride in the amount required to correct moderate depletion can be neglected. For severe sodium depletion, the amount of sodium needed may be much greater than is supplied by 3 litres of 0.9 per cent saline; for massive sodium replacement, hypertonic (5 per cent) saline has the advantages of a smaller volume of fluid actually infused, and a more rapid restoration of plasma volume and renal circulation. When patients with severe sodium depletion are given hypertonic sodium infusions, they retain less water than would be needed to dilute the infusions down to isotonicity, and commonly they do not experience the thirst which would be induced in a normal subject by the same infusion; this suggests that much of the water lost from the E.C.F. as sodium depletion develops has gone into the cells, and is available for dilution of hypertonic saline (Black, 1953; Gordillo et al, 1957). When large amounts of sodium are given, about a fifth should be in

E

combination with lactate and this can conveniently be done by adding molar lactate to the 5 per cent infusion of sodium chloride, one 40 ml ampoule to each 200 ml of saline. The amount of lactate should be modified when there is significant acidosis or alkalosis, as is common in those losses of gastric or intestinal fluids which are the most frequent causes of massive sodium depletion.

Hyponatraemic Syndromes*

Various conditions have now been described in which the plasma sodium concentration is diminished (Fuisz, 1963). A detailed classification of these syndromes has been presented by Danowski et al (1955), but they can be grouped more simply as follows:

(1) True sodium depletion (p. 49).
(2) Water intoxication (p. 34).
(3) Low plasma sodium associated with oedema resistant to diuretics, and often with extrarenal uraemia.
(4) Inappropriate secretion of A.D.H.
(5) 'New steady states.'
(6) Artificial dilution of plasma sodium by excess of glucose, fat, or protein in the plasma (p. 30, footnote).†

Only the first of these syndromes is necessarily associated with depletion of total body-sodium, though this may complicate the others on occasion, except syndrome (3), in which body-sodium is always increased as shown by the oedema.

Attention was drawn to syndrome (3) by Schroeder (1949) and it

---

* This term is used in this edition in preference to 'low salt syndromes'. Euphony and the fear of neologisms are not the only considerations in choosing words; the term now used focuses attention on sodium *concentration*, which is the resultant of several factors, and not solely dependent on the body-content of sodium, let alone of 'salt'.

† In a very informative account of the matter, Leaf (1962) groups hyponatraemia into these 3 categories: (a) 'with adequate circulation and expanded E.C.F. volume', (b) 'with circulatory insufficiency and contracted E.C.F. volume', (c) 'with circulatory insufficiency and over-expanded E.C.F. volume'. To match this descriptive classification with the one given here in terms of mechanisms, Leaf's a corresponds to my 2 and 4, Leaf's b to my 1, and Leaf's c to my 3.

has often been observed since, in association with various measures of therapeutic salt depletion.* These act in the first instance on the plasma, either by diminishing the entry of sodium from the bowel or by increasing its elimination by the kidneys. When the peripheral circulation is grossly inadequate, the plasma volume and sodium concentration may be diminished by such means, even in the presence of peripheral oedema, which is as it were functionally outside the body. The renal circulation may thus be diminished to an even greater extent than is usual in cardiac failure, and the blood urea rises to 100 mg or more per 100 ml. The relative importance of low plasma volume and of low sodium concentration in impairing renal function is difficult to assess in this particular syndrome, in which both abnormalities are present. It should be recalled, however, that in water intoxication, with even lower plasma concentrations of sodium, renal excretory function is not impaired. In his original account, Schroeder (1949) laid emphasis on the hyponatraemia, and described improvement and a fall in the blood urea when hypertonic saline was infused. A favourable response to hypertonic saline in this syndrome is, in my experience, unusual; the administered sodium often only increases the oedema without improving the circulation. There are a few patients in whom the venous pressure is low, and in them hypertonic saline is worth a trial; but most patients in this group have a raised venous pressure, and it is difficult to see how their circulation can be improved by saline infusion. Another indication for a trial of hypertonic saline in patients with congestive heart failure may be an exceptionally high blood urea for this state, e.g. above 100 mg/100 ml. The conjunction of hyponatraemia and oedema is not, of course, limited to patients with congestive failure,

* Marriott (1953) has reviewed the important part played by different forms of treatment in inducing 'iatrogenic salt depletion'. Apart from deliberate attempts at sodium depletion by low-salt diets, diuretics and exchange resins, the main causes listed are mechanical removal of fluids, intravenous therapy with non-saline fluids, ileo- and other ostomies and the 'diarrhoea medicamentosa' which may follow broad-spectrum antibiotic treatment. One might also mention the dangers of purgation in Addison's disease and thyrotoxicosis, so effectively castigated by Witts (1937) under the head of 'ritual purgation'; I have myself seen severe desiccation in a moderately uraemic patient following the use or abuse of magnesium sulphate.

but occurs also in the hypoproteinaemic oedemas. For example, Vere and King (1960) have studied in some detail the effects of withdrawing oedema fluid by acupuncture from nephrotic patients; they observed a fall in the plasma [Na] and an increase in the blood-urea level.

Schwartz et al (1960) observed three patients with bronchial neoplasm in whom hyponatraemia was due mainly to water retention, although there was also some loss of Na in the urine. The hyponatraemia persisted even when urinary salt loss was prevented by mineralocorticoids, but the plasma [Na] rose when water intake was restricted. They suggested that these findings could be explained by 'inappropriate secretion of A.D.H.', leading to water retention even when the body-fluids were dilute. The loss of Na in the urine, when present, was secondary to the increased volume of body-fluid, which would increase G.F.R. and also inhibit aldosterone secretion. Williams (1963) showed in a similar patient that aldosterone secretion was normal; so the increase in G.F.R. may be the most important factor. Another factor in producing hyponatraemia may be entry of Na into cells, as suggested by Kaye (1966). Carter et al (1961) suggest that inappropriate secretion of A.D.H. may account for the hyponatraemia sometimes associated with cerebral damage. Since expansion of volume can lead to increase in Na excretion, the current status of 'cerebral salt-wasting' is in some doubt. Nelson et al (1951) had earlier suggested that increased A.D.H. activity could be one factor in causing hyponatraemia following paracentesis in cirrhotic patients with ascites. Grumer et al (1962) have observed episodic hyponatraemia in an otherwise healthy subject, with evidence that the episodes were related to inappropriate A.D.H. secretion. There is evidence of actual neoplastic production of material with vasopressin activity in the case of bronchial neoplasm (Barraclough et al, 1966), adding another to the list of pharmacological agents derived from tumours (Greenberg et al, 1964). Bartter and Schwartz (1967) have reviewed the syndrome of inappropriate A.D.H. secretion.

Under the heading of 'new steady states', we may include a number of conditions in which the low plasma sodium seems to depend not on any alteration in the external balance of sodium, but on an altered distribution of sodium within the body. From the practical point of view, the chief characteristic of this group is that the plasma sodium cannot be increased to normal levels by hypertonic saline, and the patients are not improved, and may be made worse, by such treatment. There are patients with chronic wasting disease, notably tuberculosis, who have a low plasma sodium but no evidence of dehydration, and who show a normal excretory response to variation in salt intake (Sims *et al*, 1950). In some patients, the plasma [Na] increases when potassium is given, without change in the external Na balance; the administered K may have in part entered cells, displacing Na which had previously accumulated intracellularly (Laragh, 1954). These patients do not have an increase in plasma potassium, and they differ in this from patients with terminal disease, especially anoxic patients, who may have a low plasma sodium and raised plasma K, possibly reflecting a breakdown of the mechanisms which maintain the discrepancy in electrolyte composition between E.C.F. and I.C.F. The concept of a partial breakdown in the energy-requiring mechanisms which maintain the Na/K gradient across the cell-walls has been crystallized in the dramatic term 'sick-cell syndrome'. This is not a diagnosis to be made with ease or confidence, and is becoming less frequent with recognition of other mechanisms for hyponatraemia.

Since we have advocated hypertonic saline in the treatment of sodium depletion, and also, in small amounts, in the treatment of water intoxication, it is relevant to discuss the frequency, relative to these conditions, of the low-salt syndromes which do not respond to hypertonic saline, and which may be aggravated by its use. For this purpose, we have set out in Table 3.2 a summary of the results of Danowski *et al* (1955); this shows the relative incidence in various disease-groups of a plasma sodium less than 132 mEq/l.—an abnormality which was found in 291 analyses in a series of 6462. Results on children have been omitted from the table. This material is probably fairly representative of the findings in medical wards; among surgical patients, true sodium depletion is probably more frequent, because of losses of gastro-intestinal fluids. Admittedly, a moderate degree of hyponatraemia is very common after operations (Moore, 1954; Zimmerman *et al*, 1956); but it is not known to cause symptoms or to require treatment. In medical patients, it is interesting to note that a low plasma sodium not requiring saline is as common as true sodium depletion, and more common than water intoxication. It follows that treatment with saline should be given only when a low plasma sodium is accompanied by evidence of low

TABLE 3.2

Relative incidence of the causes of low plasma sodium

	Sodium depletion	Water intoxication	Other
Diabetes	9	6	4
G.I. tract	6	6	1
C.N.S.	2	1	—
Cardiac	3	—	4
Renal	9	3	21
Pulmonary	—	—	2
Other	2	2	1
	31	18	33

This table is a summary of the information on adult patients given in Table 4 of Danowski et al (1955). The column marked 'other' includes the categories of 'cellular hypo-osmolality' and 'new steady state', whose separation is difficult and whose significance, in respect of the need for administering sodium, is the same.

plasma or E.C.F. volume, and of a likely channel of sodium loss from the body. Although theoretically clear-cut, the decision may be difficult in practice, and then a therapeutic trial of 200 ml of 5 per cent saline is justified.

Sodium Excess

By far the most common manifestation of an excess of sodium in the body is generalized oedema; but the formation of oedema requires the retention not only of sodium and associated anions, but also of water. When water retention is prevented, sodium excess may manifest itself as an increase in the sodium concentration of plasma, without oedema. *Hypernatraemia* of moderate degree without oedema is a regular finding in water depletion (p. 33); and many of the reported instances of hypernatraemia could be due to unrecognized water depletion rather than to any absolute excess of Na in the body. For example, hypernatraemia has been found in infants whose feeds were made with insufficient water (Simpson and O'Duffy, 1967). Since hypernatraemia fundamentally expresses hyperosmolality, it can be induced by a high intake of other solutes as well as of sodium salts; a high solute/water ratio in the body can be based on urea or on glucose as well as on sodium-salts, e.g. the hypernatraemia of high-protein feeding and that found occasionally in diabetic coma (de Graeff and Lips, 1957). Actual excess of Na itself in the body in association with hypernatraemia occurs with excessive renal retention of Na, most notably in primary aldosteronism, but also in Cushing's syndrome; and with a relatively greater intake of salt than of water, a situation usually induced in severely ill people by hypertonic saline,* or in helpless infants by 'salt-poisoning', leading to 'hypernatraemic dehydration' (Harrison and Finberg, 1959). Sodium sulphate given in the treatment of hypercalcaemia has led to hypernatraemia (Heckman and Walsh, 1967). Normally, hypernatraemia is prevented by thirst and by the renal capacity to excrete urine of high solute/water ratio (see Chapter II); but Leaf (1962) has described the respect for these usual regulatory mechanisms which was instilled into him by having to look after patients who had lost both thirst and neurohypophyseal function as a result of brain tumours. Although mannitol diuresis leads to a loss of Na from the body, and the urine formed is of higher osmolality than plasma, nevertheless this osmolality is largely accounted for by the loading solute itself, and the net loss of water is greater than the net loss of Na. On such a basis, Moore (1963) predicted that prolonged mannitol diuresis might cause hypernatraemia; and this has been duly observed by Gipstein and Boyle (1965).

The effects of hypernatraemia are difficult to dissociate from those of the primary disorder and of the water depletion which generally accompanies it. Finberg and his colleagues (1963) have reported a tragedy in which the feeds of 14 infants were made up with salt

---

* This usually is given intravenously, but Ward (1963) reports a patient with hypernatraemia to whom 10 per cent NaCl had been given as an emetic; he had, however, taken a large dose of perphenazine, which prevented emesis, and the large dose (300 ml) of 10 per cent NaCl was presumably absorbed.

instead of sugar, with 6 deaths. The serum [Na] rose to over 200 mEq/l., and in one infant, who recovered, to 275 mEq/l. Treatment was with peritoneal dialysis. The symptoms were mainly related to the central nervous system—coma, hyper-reflexia, pyrexia and hyperpnœa. Brain damage of various types associated with hypernatraemia has been reported in heat-stroke (Malamud et al, 1946), and following the use of hypertonic salt in inducing abortion (Cameron and Dayan, 1966). There is some evidence that not only acute hypernatraemia of this type, but also the more chronic and moderate hypernatraemia observed in nephrogenic diabetes insipidus, can lead to mental impairment (Moncrieff, 1960), as well as to irritability, retarded growth and low-grade fever (Leaf, 1962). Gross hypernatraemia may affect cardiac function; Eliakim et al (1959) observed E.C.G. changes in dogs after infusion of 20 per cent NaCl. An interesting association of hypernatraemia is hypocalcaemia (Finberg, 1957). There is some evidence, reviewed by Dahl (1958), relating a high salt intake to an increased incidence of hypertension, but the mechanism for this association, if established, is not known.

The real challenge presented by sodium excess lies of course not in hypernatraemia, but in the various forms of oedema. The immense effort expended on this problem, apparent in the review by Moyer and Fuchs (1960), makes me hesitant in offering an eclectic summary of a few pages; if it should appear dogmatic, compression must be my excuse, and not any certainty inherent in the subject-matter. (For example, in this edition I have felt obliged to replace the bold sub-heading 'excessive aldosterone activity' by the less committed 'excessive sodium reabsorption'.)

The dietary intake of sodium plays a relatively small part in producing an excess of sodium in the body, which is primarily based on defective urinary excretion of sodium. In other words, while the sodium in the body of course comes from the diet, or exceptionally from intravenous infusion, normal renal function will quickly dispose of dietary sodium excess; it is only when the kidneys are acting abnormally on the sodium brought to them that it is allowed to accumulate in the body; and when this has happened dietary control of sodium intake is not an effective means by itself of ridding the body of sodium, for even in normal people on a low-sodium diet the renal excretion of sodium becomes vanishingly small. The essential factor in producing sodium excess is therefore a failure of the kidney to make its normal response to sodium excess in the body by excreting increased amounts of Na. This failure may arise through a number of mechanisms, which may be broadly considered under the heads of (1) intrinsic renal disease, (2) inadequate renal perfusion and (3) excessive tubular reabsorption of sodium.

(1) INTRINSIC RENAL DISEASE

It is of some practical importance to distinguish between sodium retention directly due to structural change in the kidney and sodium retention associated with such change, but mediated wholly or in part by extrarenal mechanisms. The first case is exemplified by the sodium retention of urinary suppression, the second by the oedema which may occur in chronic renal failure with hypertension, and which is really the oedema of cardiac failure. The practical bearing of this distinction is that diuretic agents are of value in 'extrarenal sodium retention', but when the sodium retention is directly related to structural renal change, diuretic agents are usually ineffective and possibly dangerous.

In theory, intrinsic renal disease could cause sodium retention either by diminishing sodium filtration, or by increasing the proportion of filtered sodium which is reabsorbed by the tubules; it is this antagonism between glomerular loss and tubular conservation of sodium which is sometimes crystallized in the term 'glomerulo-tubular imbalance'. It must be admitted, however, that sodium retention is very often absent in patients in whom destruction of glomeruli is far advanced, and is producing nitrogen retention; whereas patients with the nephrotic syndrome can be grossly oedematous because of hypoproteinaemia at a stage when their G.F.R. is still normal. In acute tubular necrosis, and to a less extent in acute nephritis, the abnormal behaviour of the tubules is associated with striking morphological changes; but the correlation of structure with this particular aspect of renal function is inconstant, and in other types of oedema the excessive reabsorption of sodium by the tubules has no apparent structural concomitant.

(2) INADEQUATE RENAL PERFUSION

In patients with oligaemic shock and also in those with acutely induced hypotension, the renal blood flow and G.F.R. are much depressed, and the excretion of sodium at this time is very low indeed. Experimentally, constriction of the renal arteries leads to sodium retention (Pitts and Duggan, 1950). Sodium retention, without heart disease or albuminuria, has been reported by Fischer *et al* (1959) as a result of massive renal arterial occlusion. Such a sequence is very exceptional, and for the most part inadequate renal perfusion is either transient or fatal; but it may play some part in the oedema of congestive heart failure. The renal blood flow and G.F.R. are substantially reduced not only in 'low-output' failure, but even in patients with a raised cardiac output in cor pulmonale (Davies and Kilpatrick, 1951; Fishman *et al*, 1951). Moreover, transient increases in renal blood flow, such as happen at night in early cardiac failure, have been associated with increases in G.F.R. and also in output of salt and water, which may be clinically evident as nocturia (Brod and Fejfar, 1950). Propranalol has been shown to induce similar loss of the diurnal rhythm in normal subjects, while in patients with heart disease it can cause outright Na retention with manifest oedema (Epstein and Braunwald, 1966). These changes in cardiac output, which have been particularly stressed by Borst (1948), are almost certainly not the entire explanation of cardiac oedema, a state whose complexity transcends the easy antithesis between 'forward' and 'backward' failure (Sodeman, 1960). The local effects of a raised venous pressure on the kidneys are also possibly of some importance, but it is becoming clear that the changes in renal circulation in cardiac failure are at least equalled in importance by an alteration in tubular handling of sodium.

(3) EXCESSIVE SODIUM REABSORPTION

In patients who are accumulating oedema-fluid, and who are not under the immediate influence of diuretics, the output of Na in the urine is vanishingly small. It is now generally agreed that depressed G.F.R. cannot fully nor always account for this; and the discovery of aldosterone has seemed to provide a good explanation for the avid tubular reabsorption of Na. Increased amounts of aldosterone have been found in oedematous patients, and it is now perhaps a question of defining the role of aldosterone in different types of oedema, rather than of establishing that it has a role. Suspicion that aldosterone is not universally concerned in the genesis of oedema is based mainly on two things—the dissimilarity between Conn's syndrome (primary aldosteronism) and the postulated state of 'secondary aldosteronism'; and some lack of constancy in the findings of increased aldosterone in oedematous patients. The hall-marks of primary aldosteronism are severe and obvious potassium-depletion, hypertension, and increase in plasma [Na], while oedema is unusual (Conn, 1955); a 'congenital' form is now suggested, with malignant hypertension as the main feature, but still without oedema (Conn, 1961). Primary aldosteronism has indeed been invoked as an explanation for episodic oedema (Mach *et al*, 1955); but this is a difficult case to establish, and not less so now that non-adrenal causes of episodic oedema are being reported, which could lead, as suggested by Greenough *et al* (1962), to secondary aldosteronism via renal ischaemia. There seems, then, to be some difficulty in identifying the effects of recognized hyper-aldosteronism with oedema; and the results of aldosterone assays in oedematous patients have not been entirely consistent, especially in cardiac oedema. Wolff *et al* (1957) observed aldosterone excretion in forty patients with cardiac failure; while increased excretion was common, and associated with Na retention, it was absent in about a third of the patients. In a very limited series of estimates of plasma-aldosterone (Wolff and Torbica, 1963) two out of four estimates in congestive failure were within the normal range, even though one of the patients was retaining Na at the time. Moreover, Laragh (1962) in six patients with cardiac failure observed aldosterone secretion rates ranging from 160–515 µg/day, which he states to be 'normal or only slightly elevated', and very much lower than those found by the same method in patients with cirrhosis and the nephrotic syndrome. There is, however, in congestive heart failure a reduced hepatic 'clearance' of aldosterone, arising both because of reduced hepatic blood-flow, and because of less complete extraction (Tait *et al*, 1965). On the other hand, Davis *et al* (1965) regards the reduced hepatic blood-flow as the major factor, and find no evidence of enzyme defect, suggested by earlier work of Yates et al (1958) on inactivation, and of Coppage et al (1962) on conjugation of aldosterone.

It is impossible to be dogmatic on the very limited figures available, but there is at least a hint that when oedema is based on protein depletion, and associated with a low plasma-volume, aldosterone activity is increased, and possibly of direct pathogenetic importance. In cardiac oedema, with normal or even increased plasma-volume, an increase in aldosterone is less constant, and may be rather a consequence of therapeutic de-salting than an integral part of the pathogenesis of the oedema. Less efficient hepatic inactivation of oestrogens and of A.D.H. have been suggested in cardiac failure. By inducing water retention, A.D.H. could contribute to hyponatraemia; but it could not be responsible for Na retention.

The well-established categories of generalized cardiac, renal and hepatic oedema are now seen to be incomplete. The hypoproteinaemic oedemas now include not only nutritional oedema, failure of hepatic synthesis of protein and massive renal loss of protein—the protein-losing kidney of Platt (1959)—but also at least two new syndromes of great interest. Gordon (1959) used ^{131}I-polyvinyl pyrrolidone to demonstrate in certain patients with 'idiopathic hypoproteinaemia' a leakage of large molecules into the gastrointestinal tract. This condition, now generally known as protein-losing gastro-enteropathy, has to be excluded in any patient with obscure oedema associated with hypoproteinaemia. A quite different observation, but of equal interest, is that after hypothermia, some patients become oedematous, and also show a focal pancreatitis, with high levels of serum-amylase (Duguid et al, 1961); it has been suggested that kallikrein, which is of pancreatic origin, may be responsible for an increase in capillary permeability (Howard et al, 1963). In conformity with this suggestion are the reports of patients with hereditary episodic oedema whose serum lacked the usual inhibitors of kallikrein (Landerman et al, 1962) or of serum C'l-esterase, another possible agent increasing capillary permeability (Donaldson and Evans, 1963). Though an increase in capillary permeability has long been recognized in inflammatory and allergic oedema, usually local, it has not been greatly considered in the generalized oedemas since the demonstration by Warren and Stead (1944), confirmed in a larger series by Crockett (1956), of a low protein content in the fluid of the common forms of generalized oedema. Using a gel-filtration method, Jones and Peters (1966) found no evidence of increased capillary permeability in patients with congestive heart failure, acute nephritis, 'nephrosis', and 'hypoproteinaemic oedema of non-renal origin'. It is true that a massive leak of protein through the capillary walls leads to shock, rather than to anasarca (Clarkson et al, 1960); but minor increase in capillary permeability may have been too easily discounted, though it has been invoked from time to time to explain unusual patterns of oedema (Ross et al, 1958; Weinbren, 1963).

The *treatment* of sodium excess brings gains which are indeed limited, in the sense that they do not affect the underlying disease process, but are still well worth while, in that they can change a bed-fast invalid into a moderately or even fully active person. It follows from this that sodium depletion can never engross the whole management of a patient, which must have as its primary aims the cure or palliation of his primary disease, and helping him to adjust to his remaining disability; but effective sodium depletion can make some patients fit for more radical treatment, and it can lessen or even abolish dyspnoea and oedema for useful periods in patients with irrecoverable disease. In the spectrum of palliative agents, diuretics come somewhere between insulin or cyanocobalamin on the one hand, and aminopterine or ionizing radiations on the other.

The effective agents currently in use for achieving sodium depletion act in one of three ways—by decreasing effective intake, by increasing renal elimination, or by directly removing oedema-fluid or transudates with their contained sodium. Sweating and purging are no longer in repute, and the artificial kidney is limited in value by practical considerations, though those models with a supported membrane are quite efficient in ultrafiltration of fluid from the body. Fluid can also be effectively removed from the body by peritoneal dialysis with hyperosmolar solutions. Methods of sodium depletion are often combined, and it is only for descriptive purposes that we separate them now.

(a) *Restriction of intake.* Most of the sodium in a normal diet has been added to the raw food in the form of sodium chloride either as a preservative or as a condiment; the remainder represents the natural sodium content of animal and plant tissues. By avoiding the addition of salt in cooking and at table a reasonable diet can be devised with a salt content of about 3 g/day, corresponding to 50 mEq of Na. Most of the remaining salt in the diet is in bread, and by the use of special salt-free bread the intake can be got down to 1 g of salt or about 20 mEq of Na daily; and the food is still recognizable as such. A Kempner rice-fruit diet is practically free of sodium (less than 10 mEq/day), but is is deficient in protein and in palatability. The essential difficulties in effecting sodium depletion by diet arise from the monotony of really low-sodium diets; from the uncooperative way in which the kidneys promptly lower their sodium output to match the intake; and from the practical problems which the preparation of this type of diet entails outside hospital. In this country at least, most patients settle for a mixed diet with no added salt, providing about 50 mEq of Na, and more vigorous salt depletion must be sought by other means. Before this Laodicean policy is condemned outright, it should be recalled that prolonged rigorous dietary restriction of any kind has its dangers; the special risks of low-sodium diets, and the dietetic problems created, have been fully treated in a National Research Council publication (1954).

A hopeful approach to extreme sodium restriction without complete dietary distortion lies in the use of cation exchange resins; this application was suggested by Dock (1946). Early difficulties with granular resins in the hydrogen cycle, which caused considerable local irritation and dyspepsia, have now been largely surmounted with resins in the ammonium and potassium cycles which are available as impalpable powders; but other troubles persist which will probably not be resolved unless resins can be devised with a specific affinity for sodium. Long-continued use of resins is practicable (Rosenheim and Spencer, 1956); but it requires close biochemical control, for acidosis, potassium depletion or excess, and depletion of calcium, magnesium and iron have all been met with. In the upper alimentary tract, whose secretions are of high sodium content, effective uptake of sodium takes place, but this is largely exchanged again for potassium in the colon (Spencer et al, 1954). Even the best of resins falls short of being a welcome food; and they are now little used in the treatment of oedema, since the advent of effective oral diuretics.

(b) *Increase of urinary sodium output.* In the treatment of oedema, an effective diuresis is one which lessens the amount of Na in the body; this done, the requisite changes in body-content of chloride, bicarbonate, and water will follow. In achieving natriuresis, general measures such as bed-rest, transfusion and digitalization may play an important part; and in assessing the effects of formal diuretic agents it is important to control the effect of such general measures by some form of alternating scheme such as that devised by Gold *et viii al* (1960). In comparing diuretics A and B, the patient is allowed a few days of general treatment, and when the urinary output of Na is reasonably stable, the diuretics are given in the order ABBA, BAAB with a day *off* diuretic treatment separating each day *on* diuretic treatment. The efficiency of diuretic agents is assessed by their effect on Na output, and in the long term on the patient's weight; but a complete assessment comprises side-actions as well as effectiveness, so other electrolytes as well as Na have to be estimated in plasma and urine. It would be Utopian to expect every physician to carry out a trial on a new diuretic before using it, but he should find out whether such a trial has been done; when the established diuretics fail, it is usually because of grossly inadequate filtration of sodium, or because of secondary effects of the diuretics already given, and *not* because the diuretic is less than the latest available. Diuretics have made an immense contribution to the comfort and survival of patients with cardiac failure (left and/or right) and with other forms of oedema; and the introduction of effective oral diuretics has made these benefits more practically available. The principles underlying diuretic treatment are reviewed by Pitts (1959), and many of the applications are discussed in Moyer and Fuchs (1960). We are indebted to Wilson (1963) in his Bradshaw lecture for a most able blending of theory and practice, and felicity in his account of the therapeutic aspects. He has since placed us further in his debt by a detailed account of diuretics currently in use (Lant and Wilson, 1967). Here, I can only hope to categorize the main agents by which natriuresis can be achieved.

(1) *Increase in the amount of Na filtered* at the glomerulus, and so potentially available for excretion, is obtained when the cardiac output is increased, or when renal vasospasm is relaxed. This is exemplified by the natriuresis which may follow transfusion (Borst, 1948); and also by the action of the xanthine diuretics such as aminophylline which are renal vasodilators, as well as general antispasmodics.

(2) Measures which *increase the plasma protein concentration* in the hypoproteinaemic oedemas, e.g. albumin infusions, or the effect of steroids in diminishing albuminuria in some patients with the nephrotic syndrome. There is probably a dual action here—expanding the plasma-volume improves the cardiac output and so the renal blood-flow; and also lessens the volume stimulus to aldosterone secretion.

(3) *Osmotic diuretics.* By their presence in the lumen of the tubule, these agents restrain the reabsorption of fluid, including sodium. Urea is likely to have a purely renal action, but diuretics of high molecular weight, such as mannitol and dextran may facilitate diuresis by their extrarenal action as plasma-expanders.

(4) *Inhibitors of active tubular transport.* This group contains the really effective pharmacological diuretics, notably the mercurials and the chlorothiazide derivatives. In spite of much effort, there is still no certainty which enzyme system is interfered with by these agents; although the chlorothiazide series are akin to agents such as acetazolamide, which are strong inhibitors of carbonic anhydrase, the most potent natriuretics in the group have little or no action on carbonic anhydrase. Nor do we know their site of action in the nephron, though perhaps the balance of evidence favours a 'more proximal' rather than a 'more distal' site, at least for the thiazides.

For practical purposes, the *mercurials* have to be given by intramuscular injection. Intravenous administration has caused fatalities, and the oral and subcutaneous preparations are not satisfactory. In spite of the inconvenience of injection, the mercurials are rapid and effective in an emergency, and are a good choice in established cardiac failure in hospital. There is commonly relatively greater excretion of Cl than of Na, so ammonium chloride should be given with mercurials, unless contraindicated by acidosis or hepatic insufficiency; it has to be given in a form which the patient can absorb. If ammonium chloride is not effectively given, an alkalosis may develop in patients given mercurials, and this is one mechanism whereby the diuretic loses its effect (Schwartz and Wallace, 1951); the situation is recognized by estimating plasma [H] and [HCO$_3$], and corrected by ammonium chloride or arginine chloride (Mizgala et al, 1963). Another remediable situation of mercurial resistance is that in which forced chloruresis together with a low-salt diet have led to the excretion of K instead of Na; this can be dealt with by giving KCl. If the filtration of Na is too low, not even mercurials can cause a diuresis.

While mercurials hold their value for the acute situation, their inconvenience makes them less suitable for .ong-term maintenance, and hence the *thiazides* represent a major advance, being effective oral agents, with few side-actions. More potent derivatives than the original chlorothiazide, e.g. hydrochlorothiazide, hydroflumethiazide, bendrofluazide, are given in smaller dosage; but the family resemblance is strong, including occasional sensitization with skin-rashes and thrombocytopenia. They all have a tendency to induce K depletion, and attempts to differentiate between them on this score are mainly of commercial interest.* It is better to add a K supplement, whose dose can be varied, than to use tablets with a fixed amount of K. A further considerable argument against incorporating a potassium salt in diuretic tablets is the ulceration of the bowel which can be induced by concentrated potassium salts applied locally (Baker et al, 1964). Supplementation with K is specially necessary in cardiac patients who are taking digitalis, because of the possible insidious potentation of the toxic effects of digitalis (see p. 84). The thiazides have useful side-actions as mild hypotensives; and as antagonists of water losing in diabetes insipidus (including the nephrogenic disorder). They may, however, lead to a rise in blood-sugar, or in plasma-urate, generally subclinical, but occasionally associated with frank diabetes or gout.

An oral diuretic which has been shown to be effective is triamterene (Baba et al, 1962), which has a different mode of action, and

---

* It is remarkable what manufacturers, unfettered by evidence, will claim for their products; for example, chlorthalidone (Hygroton) is recommended on the grounds that its action lasts for over 24 hours—an 'advantage' which most people would be prepared to forego in a diuretic.

F

may therefore supplement the thiazides; but has the disadvantage of causing nitrogen retention. The most rapidly-acting and potent diuretics in current use are ethacrynic acid (Melvin et al, 1963), and frusemide (Forrester and Shirriffs, 1965). These qualities give them value in the treatment of critical left-ventricular failure, or of oedema which has resisted other diuretics. Their brisk action also increases the risk of those side-effects, such as hypovolaemia and hyponatraemia, which are the result of too-rapid discharge of Na. The moderate thiazides are at present the drugs of choice for the regular care of oedematous patients, the more potent drugs being held in reserve.

(5) *Aldosterone antagonists.* Metyrapone inhibits the synthesis of aldosterone, as well as of cortisol; while the spirolactones antagonize the action of aldosterone on the distal tubule. In strict logic, this group should be reserved for those patients in whom an excessive secretion of aldosterone is an important part of the mechanism of oedema formation, e.g. in hypoproteinaemia. However, since a moiety of Na-reabsorption is probably attributable to aldosterone even in normal people, some natriuretic action is to be expected in oedema generally, especially as the low-salt diet will promote an increased aldosterone secretion. In conjunction with the thiazides, spironolactone has the advantages that it lowers K excretion, and that it could lessen reabsorption in the distal tubule of Na coming down from the proximal tubule under the action of the thiazide (Edmonds, 1960). But we do not yet know all the actions either of aldosterone or of its antagonists; and it seems safer to reserve these for trial in those patients not readily controlled by other means.

In resistant oedema, a combination of agents is often necessary. The combination of an osmotic diuretic (mannitol), chlorothiazide, and an aldosterone-inhibitor, although exacting for the patient, has been shown to be effective in treating resistant ascites when other measures have failed (Shaldon et al, 1960). Corticosteroids have been observed to produce a definite, but probably not practically useful, increase in Na output in intractable oedema (Bayliss, 1966).

(c) *Direct removal of E.C.F.* Removal of pleural and peritoneal transudates is primarily carried out to relieve dyspnoea or abdominal discomfort, and the loss of sodium from the body is incidental. The amount of fluid removed from the chest is seldom sufficient to cause acute sodium depletion, but massive drainage of ascitic fluid may lead to oligaemic shock from loss of protein and extracellular electrolyte. Subcutaneous drainage by Southey's tubes fell into disuse because of the frequency of septic complications, but has been revived by the introduction of more effective drainage tubes and the use of antibiotics. The patient should have as much fluid as possible drained by gravity into his legs, and surprisingly large amounts of fluid can then be obtained. The result may, however, be disappointing when the oedema is long-standing and complicated by induration; and the method is now much less used than it was say five years ago.

The practice of sodium depletion cannot be summarized in a few words. The basic weapons available are a diet moderately restricted in sodium content and the use either of intramuscular mercurial diuretics at first on alternate days and later once or twice weekly, or of an efficient oral diuretic of the chlorothiazide series. The selection of other measures when these fail or become less effective is often difficult, and should be preceded by an analysis of plasma for Na, K, Cl, HCO_3 and urea. This may give a lead to some simple measure such as giving ammonium or potassium chloride, or exchange-resin in small doses, which will restore the diuretic response. In cases of unusually resistant oedema, the addition of an osmotic diuretic and/or an aldosterone antagonist may meet the difficulty. If the problem is one of sensitivity to the thiazides, then a drug of another series should be used, e.g. frusemide or ethacrynic acid.

Let me stress once again that the use of diuretics is by no means limited to patients with overt peripheral oedema. They have a dramatic action in paroxysmal nocturnal dyspnoea, and are helpful in left-ventricular failure in general—and also, it has been claimed, in patients with respiratory failure (Noble et al, 1966). The thiazide diuretics have an ancillary function in the treatment of hypertension and of diabetes insipidus.

CHAPTER IV

POTASSIUM

Amount and Distribution

As with sodium, information is scanty on the total potassium content of the body, as determined by analysis of the cadaver. Shohl (1939) gives a mean value from the older literature of 54.8 mEq/kg body-weight, and 66.8 mEq/kg fat-free weight. More recent values on non-oedematous adults are shown in Table 4.1:

TABLE 4.1

Subject	Age	Sex	Potassium content mEq/kg total wt.	mEq/kg fat free wt.
'1951'	46	♂	54.4	66.5*
'1953'	60	♂	48.6	66.6*
'L'	42	♀	55.5	72.6†
'M'	25	♂	60.8	71.3†

These figures once more bring out the relative constancy of mineral composition of the lean body mass, and the variation introduced by obesity. They are of much the same order as estimates of (K) based on the naturally-occurring long-life isotope ^{40}K. For clinical measurement of exchangeable K, however, the short-life isotope ^{42}K is generally used, and this gives results lower by some 15 per cent. In view of the correspondence between the analytical and the ^{40}K values, it seems likely that the ^{42}K values are systematically an underestimate. This could arise because equilibration was not complete within the time available; and studies of the distribution of ^{42}K in

* Forbes and Lewis (1956).   † Widdowson et al (1951).

various tissues do suggest incomplete equilibrium, certainly at 24 hours, and possibly even at 48 hours after administration of the tracer (Gowenlock *et al*, 1960). Table 4.2 gives comparative results for ^{40}K and ^{42}K in men and women; the lower values in women are probably accounted for by their higher content of fat, and consequent lower content of lean tissue.

TABLE 4.2

Method	Men	Women	References
	Potassium content of body (mEq/kg)		
^{42}K	48.1	38.2	Widdowson and Dickerson (1964)
^{40}K	55	49	Barter and Forbes (1963)

Since potassium is the predominant cation of cells, its distribution among the organs of the body is related to their cell-mass. On this

TABLE 4.3

Potassium and sodium content of various organs of man. Values are subject to considerable variation, especially in association with alterations in content of fat.

	Weight kg	K mEq	Na mEq
Whole body	70	3800	5100
Skeletal muscle	30	2730	810
Skin	18	360	1600
Erythrocytes	2.4	252	36
Bone	12	218	1600
Brain	1.9	150	133
Liver	1.8	135	74
Heart	0.3	24	11
Kidneys	0.3	18	22
Plasma	2.6	12	363

(This table is Table I of Mudge (1953). I am indebted to Dr Mudge for permission to reproduce it.)

basis, about 70 per cent of the potassium in the body is in the muscle, about 10 per cent in the skin and subcutaneous tissues, and most of the remainder in the brain and large viscera. Some of the differences in the distribution of Na and K among organs are given in Table 4.3,

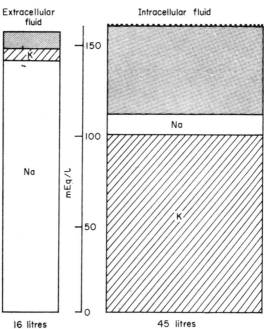

FIG. 4.1. Partition of Na and K between E.C.F. and I.C.F. Concentrations on the ordinate; volume of fluid on the abscissa, so that areas represent total amounts of Na and K. (See pp. 12, 39, 75.)

taken from Mudge (1953). The concentration of Na in E.C.F. and of K in I.C.F. of the various tissues is of the same order; so these differences largely reflect the different cellularity of the organs. The predominantly extracellular position of Na, and the intracellular position of K are summarized in Fig. 4.1.

Potassium Homeostasis

The problem of potassium homeostasis is in one way more complicated than that of sodium. Whereas the greater part of exchangeable body-sodium is in the extracellular fluid, and so accessible via the plasma to the organs of absorption and excretion, the great bulk of body K is intracellular, so that absorption and excretion are at a remove from the major K mass. In addition, there are in places collections of fluid with a [K] much higher than that of E.C.F., but lower than that of I.C.F. For example, Erulkar and Maren (1961) have shown a [K] averaging 67 mEq/l. in the fluid of the inner ear. There is a high content of carbonic anhydrase in the inner ear, and the inhibitor acetazoleamide lowers the [K] in endolymph to 15 mEq/l. There are no doubt a number of special local mechanisms of this kind; but in general we have to consider (1) the maintenance of total-body K, and (2) the regulation of E.C.F. [K].

(1) EXTERNAL BALANCE OF POTASSIUM

The daily intake of potassium on a normal diet ranges from 50–150 mEq. About 5–10 mEq of potassium are excreted in the stools, i.e. a higher proportion of the intake than for sodium. The faecal potassium probably does not represent unabsorbed dietary potassium, but rather potassium entering the colon by ion-exchange for Na which is being reabsorbed (Berger, 1960). Only small amounts of K are excreted in the sweat, though the proportion of K to Na increases under the influence of adrenal mineralocorticoids. However, Tinckler (1966) has shown that in the tropics loss of K in the sweat may be of the same order as that of Na. The precise regulation of potassium balance rests with the kidneys, which respond to high intake by increased excretion, and to low intake by conservation of potassium to the extent of producing urine with a [K] lower than that of plasma (Fourman, 1954a). There is a diurnal rhythm of potassium excretion analogous to that of sodium, and also under most circumstances roughly coincident with the sodium rhythm. However, when ostensible time is abruptly altered, as by flying the Atlantic, the sodium rhythm accommodates itself to the new situation in a day or two, whereas that for potassium takes some days longer. Diurnal rhythms in man, under their synthetic name 'circadian' (from *circa* and *dies*) are reviewed by Mills (1966).

On a moderate intake of K, the urinary excretion of K is about 70 μEq/min; at a plasma level of 5 mEq/l. of K, and a G.F.R. of

100 ml/min, the amount of K filtered is 500 μEq/min. This behaviour could quite well be accounted for by the failure of some 15 per cent of the filtered potassium to be reabsorbed in the tubules. However, in renal failure, and on a high K intake in normal people, it has been observed that excreted K may exceed filtered K. This indicates tubular secretion of K, and there is now considerable evidence that this process is not limited to the special circumstances in which it is easily demonstrable, but is the mechanism by which urinary K is normally excreted. For example, Berliner *et al* (1951) showed that the excretion of K and H ions were related in such a way as to suggest that they shared a common path of exchange for reabsorbed Na; since the glomerular filtrate contains no significant amount of H ions, these must be secreted, and their relationship to excreted K suggests that this also is secreted. The same group have also shown that moderate depression of G.F.R. does not lower the excretion of K, suggesting that filtered K does not constitute any large part of the K ultimately excreted (Davidson *et al*, 1957). In microcatheterization studies, Hierholzer (1961) found evidence that in the hamster the secretion of K took place in the accessible collecting ducts, but that there must also be some secretion proximal to this. Black and Emery (1957) have reviewed the evidence for secretion of K, and have added further evidence, based on studies with ^{42}K, that urinary K is not directly derived from filtered K, but resembles K already present in the renal cells.*

(2) POTASSIUM CONCENTRATION IN E.C.F.

Even if E.C.F. [K], or rather plasma [K], may not be the determinant of K excretion, its regulation remains of importance, because of the profound effects of any large change in E.C.F. [K] on neuromuscular function. In normal subjects, 80 per cent of estimates of plasma [K]

---

* The hypothesis that filtered K is totally reabsorbed, and that K is then secreted into the final urine, may offend against the dogma 'Natura enim simplex est'; but before setting on it with Occam's familiar razor, the critic might reflect that it ascribes to urinary K an intracellular rather than an extracellular source, and so relates K excretion more directly to the characteristic situation of potassium. There is evidence that in K depletion renal cells show changes in K concentration similar to those of other tissues; so that a regulation of K excretion based on renal-cell [K] would not be far divorced from the general state of K balance.

fall between 3.9 and 5.0 mEq/l., and 98 per cent between 3.5 and 5.6 mEq/l. (Wootton and King, 1953). This range is somewhat wider, in relation to the mean value, than the corresponding range for plasma [Na]. Nevertheless, it is quite narrow in absolute terms, in view of the fact that E.C.F. is separated from a fluid of 20-fold higher concentration of K by a membrane which permits the passage of potassium very freely (Black *et al*, 1955). The plasma [K] is affected by a number of factors, which include the following:

(1) *Changes in the external balance of potassium*. Our information on this comes mainly from observations on clinical and experimental potassium depletion. Low levels of plasma [K] are commonly, but by no means invariably, found in patients depleted of potassium. In experimental K depletion, Black and Milne (1952) found a lowering of plasma [K], such that the level of [K] was correlated inversely with the magnitude of the induced K deficit; on the other hand, Lowe (1953) found normal plasma [K] with comparable total K deficits. The explanation of this discrepancy probably lies in the high Na intake of the subjects of Black and Milne, whereas Lowe used a diet free of Na as well as of K. There is less information on the effects of a high K intake, but an increase in plasma [K] can be induced by oral or parenteral administration of K, especially if the urine output is low; but most of the K load which is not excreted is accommodated within the cells.

(2) *Changes in sodium balance*. It has been known for some time that the administration of large amounts of sodium will induce a negative K balance (Bunge, 1873; Gamble, 1951), the excreted K being derived from cells. The net effect of this on plasma [K] is variable: on the one hand, K is displaced from cells by Na, which will tend to raise the plasma [K]; on the other hand, increased excretion of K and expansion of E.C.F. volume tend to lower the plasma [K]. Clinical states of sodium excess are further complicated by factors such as increased excretion of K in response to diuretics, and deficient intake from anorexia; as a general rule, the plasma [K] is normal or low in clinical sodium excess. Conversely, in severe sodium depletion, the plasma [K] is often high in spite of concurrent K depletion; this is found in patients with diabetic coma who are depleted of both Na and K, and who also have an acidosis and impaired cellular

uptake of glucose. An additional factor is the increased rate of tissue breakdown which occurs in Na depletion; this leads to the discharge of more K into the E.C.F. Of the two opposing effects on plasma [K] of change in Na balance—change in E.C.F. volume, and replacement of cellular K by Na—it is probably the former which is the more important in determining the resultant plasma [K], which therefore is often lowered in generalized oedema, and raised in severe sodium depletion.

(3) *Acidosis and alkalosis.* Acidosis increases the plasma [K], and probably does so by both renal and extrarenal mechanisms. On the Berliner mechanism (p. 78), an increased secretion of H ions would depress the secretion of K ions, leading to K retention. Much of the retained K would, however, be taken up into cells, were it not that acidosis affects the balance between intracellular and extracellular K directly, increasing the amount of K outside the cell. This phenomenon is demonstrable *in vitro*, and has also been established in nephrectomized animals by Keating *et al* (1953). It is observed in both metabolic and respiratory acidosis, and presumably represents a participation in the buffering of an acidosis by intracellular cation, which is predominantly potassium. Conversely, alkalosis whether respiratory or metabolic is associated with lowering of the plasma [K].

These effects of acidosis and alkalosis on the plasma [K] are not without clinical relevance. The clinical effects of K depletion with a low plasma [K] have been noted to be more severe when it is complicated by acidosis (Black, 1953). This may be related not only to a direct potentiation of paresis by acidosis (Lehmann, 1937), but also to the effect of acidosis in leaching K out of the cells; this will both aggravate the intracellular K depletion, and disguise its true severity, in so far as this is inferred from the plasma [K] level. In conditions of K excess, the toxic effects are largely those of a raised plasma [K]; and acidosis may then be material in aggravating this—a situation which can arise in respiratory failure with hypercapnia and a diminished renal excretion of K. In calculous oliguria with uraemia and a high plasma [K], cardiac irregularity has been observed when hypercapnia complicated anaesthesia.

(4) *Changes in cell metabolism.* The most familiar deviation of

plasma [K] induced by metabolic change is the fall in plasma [K] (and in K excretion) which attends the cellular uptake of glucose. A fall of plasma [K] takes place during a glucose tolerance test, but is sufficient to cause symptoms only if absorption of the glucose is unusually rapid, e.g. after a gastrectomy, or if the plasma [K] is already low, in which event a carbohydrate load may precipitate an attack of paresis (Milne et al, 1952). As the glycogen stores are repleted during recovery from diabetic coma, K enters cells and this may contribute to the fall in plasma [K] which may manifest itself by paresis at this stage.

Protein anabolism is also associated with cellular uptake of K, but not at a rate which sensibly diminishes the plasma level. On the other hand, the rapid protein catabolism associated with trauma, infection, tissue ischaemia and anoxia, may increase the plasma [K], though rarely to toxic levels. Breakdown of protein is not, however, the entire explanation of K loss from cells in these conditions, for the loss of K exceeds the amount corresponding to the loss of N, on the basis of the K:N ratio in tissue (in general terms, 2.7 mEq of K are associated in tissue with 1 g of N). Besides actual breakdown of protein, loss of intracellular fluid would lead to K loss from cells, and so would inefficiency of the energy metabolism on which the maintenance of intracellular-extracellular gradients of K and Na must depend. Alteration in potassium balance and distribution is only one facet of a general response to injury (see Chapter VI).

In contrast to these universal shifts of K between cells and E.C.F. in association with metabolic activity, there is the special case of familial periodic palsy, in which the episodes of paralysis are associated with transient falls in the plasma [K]. Although the attacks can be successfully treated by oral potassium, they are not related to deficit of total-body K, but to a temporary shift of K from E.C.F. into cells (Danowski et al, 1948). It has now been shown that before an attack the uptake of K into muscle is increased (Zierler and Andres, 1957), and that this process is one of the many which are subject to diurnal variation (Andres et al, 1957). Conn et al (1957) suggested that abnormally high intracellular [Na] might be more closely related to muscle function than the changes in K; and they found fluctuations in aldosterone output compatible with retention of Na preceding the paralytic attacks. On the other hand, Jones *et al* (1959) and Doak and Eyre (1961) failed to find any constant relation between paralysis and either Na retention or increase in aldosterone. The observations that paralysis can occur in some patients with normal [K] in serum (Tyler *et al*, 1951) and in others as the [K] is raised by oral potassium (van't Hoff, 1962) serve to remind us that familial periodic paralysis is not a single entity, and to suggest perhaps that intracellular events are more critical than changes in electrolyte concentration in E.C.F.

(5) *Miscellaneous factors.* Since metabolic changes influence the plasma [K], it is not surprising that a number of hormones and drugs can affect the plasma [K]. The plasma [K] is lowered by insulin, and also by adrenaline, though with adrenaline there may be a transient increase in [K] as liver glycogen is broken down. Excretion of K is increased by adrenal mineralocorticoids, and to a less extent by glucocorticoids. Bartter and Fourman (1957) have shown that with DCA the plasma [K] falls, suggesting a predominantly renal effect; while with hydrocortisone the plasma [K] is increased, suggesting that the primary change is release of K from cells into E.C.F. However, Bagshawe *et al* (1965) have observed that the prolonged administration of hydrocortisone is associated with hypokalaemia, which might be related, however, to concomitant alkalosis (Tashima, 1965). Mills *et al* (1960) observed a kaluretic effect of cortisol, not accounted for by change in plasma level; this could represent a stimulant effect of cortisol on K secretion, which in varying circumstances could lead either to Na retention in exchange, or to lessened hydrion secretion. Increase in plasma [K] has been reported with large doses of vasopressin and of thyroid extract; with histamine, acetylcholine and tyramine; and, of course, with foods and medicines rich in potassium, and exchange-resins in the potassium cycle.

Many of the clinical effects of potassium depletion and excess can be related to the changes in plasma [K]; but the foregoing account of mechanisms may have shown that while K depletion predisposes to hypokalaemia, the two states can be dissociated; and likewise K excess and hyperkalaemia. The possible dissociation of the balance and the plasma level of potassium does need some emphasis, as it may influence treatment. We shall therefore discuss some aspects of hypokalaemia in advance of the general discussion on potassium depletion.

Hypokalaemia*

Most of the recognized clinical associations of hypokalaemia were foreshadowed in the observations of Ringer (1883) that in a medium or abnormally low [K] the beats of the frog heart weakened, and finally stopped with the heart in diastole.† Both cardiac and skeletal muscle may be affected in hypokalaemia, the effects on each being somewhat variable and not rigidly associated with any set degree of hypokalaemia. This is scarcely surprising in view of the effect of other ions on muscular action, and the importance of intracellular K as well as of extracellular K.

Cardiac changes associated with hypokalaemia. Although the important relationship between cardiac function and potassium was first made manifest through experimentally induced changes in the extracellular medium, the recent work has tended to lay more emphasis on intracellular changes. At the clinical level, the E.C.F. and I.C.F. changes are difficult to dissociate, and in this section it seems better to give a general outline of the relations between K and cardiac action, rather than split it into two parts on a somewhat uncertain basis. Some patients with hypokalaemia have clinically obvious arrhythmias, tachycardia, or hypotension. There are also well-recognized but quite varied cardiographic accompaniments of hypokalaemia, reviewed by Bellet (1955), Goodwin (1958) and Swales (1964). These include ST depression with prolonged QT and a prominent U wave; T wave inversion; and the appearance of a large or even a bifid U wave in an otherwise normal tracing. There is also abundant evidence from experimental work that the cardiac muscle in K depletion shares in the intracellular loss of K, and is the seat of morphological changes, with necrosis and disruption of fibres. The relationship

---

* 'Hypokalaemia' is preferred to its popular rival 'hypopotassaemia'. Not only is it less offensive to the ear, but it does not beguile the fancy with thoughts of a bizarre zoological infestation of the blood.

† Although Ringer's description suggests that the arrested heart was dilated, later work on the mammalian heart indicates arrest in systole.

between K depletion and cardiac action is given very special clinical importance by the increasing evidence that the effects of K depletion and of digitalis, even in therapeutic dosage, are additive (Lown and Levine, 1958) and lead to the very characteristic clinical syndrome of paroxysmal atrial tachycardia with variable artio-ventricular block* (Oram *et al*, 1960; Harris *et al*, 1960).

A reasonable basis for this association can be found in the pharmacological studies reviewed by Hajdu and Leonard (1960). The resting membrane potential is a direct function of the natural logarithm of the ratio $[K]_i/[K]_e$, while the action potential is associated with brisk efflux of a tiny quantum of intracellular K. The 'irritability' of muscle varies in the same direction as membrane potential. A fall in intracellular total-potassium also increases the contractile power; this is well shown in the staircase phenomenon, in which increments of power are associated with the step-wise decrements of intracellular potassium which occur on repeated stimulation. Digitalis and other cardiac glycosides lead to a fall in (K), and so of course does substantial potassium depletion. On this basis, potassium could relate to cardiac action in 4 ways:

(1) An acute and primary fall in $[K]_e$ would increase the $[K]_i/[K]_e$ ratio, and so the irritability of muscle.

(2) Predominantly intracellular K depletion would decrease the $[K]_i/[K]_e$ ratio, and so decrease irritability.

(3) The decrement in total K_i, common both to K depletion and to digitalis action, would improve contractile power.

(4) Advanced K depletion disorganizes the whole contractile mechanism, even producing muscle disruption.

This is complicated, but so are the facts which call for explanation. For example, although P.A.T.B. was clearly associated with K depletion, and alleviated by K replacement, the majority of patients had serum [K] in the normal range (Oram *et al*, 1960). Conversely, E.C.F. [K] cannot simply be dismissed in favour of I.C.F. [K], for the *onset* of kaliopenic arrhythmia has been observed during the infusion of solutions containing both glucose and potassium, whose effect is

---

* The justification for abbreviating the name of this syndrome to P.A.T.B. is stronger than in many other instances, and we henceforth use the abbreviation.

presumably to add to total K, but also to move the added K preferentially out of E.C.F. into cells (Kunin *et al*, 1962). Again, atrioventricular block can be induced by smaller amounts of K in digitalized than in normal dogs (Fisch *et al*, 1960). There is a complicated relation between irritability of natural and ectopic foci, conductivity of bundle-tissue, and contractile power, all of which are affected by digitalis, and possibly by K depletion; this may well account for the variation in E.C.G. and clinical findings in patients affected by digitalis and K depletion. There is evidence that the giving of potassium along with insulin and glucose to patients with recent myocardial infarction, as originally advocated by Sodi-Pollares, can diminish the duration and danger of arrhythmia (Mittra, 1965).

Other changes associated with hypokalaemia. Weakness of skeletal muscle even apart from the special case of periodic paralysis has also been observed in association with hypokalaemia; and it can be corrected by amounts of potassium which raise the plasma [K], but fall far short of complete repair of a potassium deficit. Moreover, the occurrence of hypokalaemic palsy without any total K deficit is established in the familial syndrome. Again, there is no constancy of symptoms for any given level of [K]; and the palsy ranges from slight weakness of grip through widespread palsy with areflexia to a generalized paralysis with respiratory involvement and 'fish-mouth' breathing. In patients with a low plasma [Ca] and [K], correction of hypokalaemia in isolation has been attended by the appearance of tetany (Engel *et al*, 1949); and the pH of plasma also influences the effect of low [K] on muscle. Paradoxically, tetany has been observed in apparently uncomplicated K depletion with hypokalaemia; and coarse muscular twitching has also been seen. Fourman (1954b) considers that the tetany of K depletion is related to intracellular ionic distortion, and not to any particular group of E.C.F. changes.

There are obvious difficulties in defining the clinical effects of hypokalaemia *per se*, as opposed to those of cellular K depletion or of the accompanying illness. Surawicz *et al* (1957) approached this problem by infusing amounts of K sufficient to raise the plasma [K], but not to correct intracellular K depletion to any great extent. Manifestations which disappeared under these conditions could tentatively be ascribed to hypokalaemia. They included mental confusion, abdominal distension, low blood-pressure and shallow rapid breathing.

Potassium Depletion

Experimental Studies. It is possible in man by rigidly restricting the intake of potassium to achieve a moderate degree of K depletion before renal conservation of K prevents further loss; several such studies have been reported.* By the use of an acidifying resin, Fourman (1954a) induced a larger depletion in man, since some K was abstracted directly by the resin, and the acidosis also maintained urinary K at a higher level. Our knowledge of severe experimental K depletion and of the morbid anatomy is mainly based on animal experiment (Darrow, 1950; Follis *et al*, 1941); but an important addition to our knowledge of the effects of relatively uncomplicated severe K depletion in man has come from observations on patients in whom the abuse of laxatives has led to massive K depletion in the absence of notable organic disease (Schwartz and Relman, 1953).

Moderate K depletion, up to 300 mEq or less than 10 per cent of total-body K, produces no symptoms in healthy subjects. The urinary output of K falls to 10 mEq/day or less, but the time taken to achieve effective renal conservation of K is greater than in comparable experiments with Na depletion. Low plasma [K] and a metabolic alkalosis were observed by Black and Milne (1952); but these findings were absent in other subjects. Moore *et al* (1955) point out that a high intake of Na is required for the appearance of hypokalaemia and alkalosis at this level of K depletion; and they suggest that on an alkalinizing diet the alkalosis will promote hypokalaemia by retaining more K within cells. The mechanism by which 'hypokalaemic alkalosis' is produced is discussed in Chapter V. The losses of K from the body exceed the total E.C.F. potassium, and must therefore come in large part from the cells; but in general no evidence of disturbed cellular function has been established at this level of K depletion. An exception to this general statement, however, is found

---

* Black and Milne (1952); Blahd and Bassett (1953); Moore *et al* (1955); Reiner *et al* (1951); Squires *et al* (1959)

in the response of renal tubular cells to an acidosis induced by ammonium chloride (Clarke et al, 1955). In moderate K depletion, there was a failure to lower the urinary pH by the normal amount, and this was due to a decreased output of titratable acid, ammonia formation being normal. (It is interesting to compare this behaviour with that in subjects depleted of a comparable amount of Na; here titratable acid is normally formed, but ammonia formation is impaired, and this may be due to diminished renal blood flow, with consequent restriction of available glutamine—Clarke et al, 1955.) There is also, in K depletion, an abnormal response to systemic alkalosis, indicated by a persistently acid urine in the presence of 'hypokalaemic alkalosis'. One factor in causing this may be an enhanced reabsorption of bicarbonate in the proximal tubule, related to increased secretion of hydrion in that site (Rector et al, 1964). When sodium is available in the diet, the E.C.F. volume increases, so that weight may remain constant, or even increase, in spite of shrinkage of I.C.F. induced by moderate K depletion.

More severe K depletion, between 10 and 30 per cent of total-body K, has been induced by Fourman (1954a). His subjects had very definite symptoms, which included muscle-weakness, apathy and irritability, intolerance to cold, anorexia, thirst. Tetany and oedema were also observed, and the E.C.G. showed U waves. There was partial relief of some of these symptoms when the acidosis and Na depletion induced by the resin were allowed to recover, although the deficit of K had not yet been corrected.

When still greater amounts than 30 per cent of the total K are removed from the body, there is evidence of widespread damage to cell function, and the animals die with characteristic alterations both in tissue composition and in histology. This abrupt deterioration as K depletion increases may be related to the effect of the potassium contained in a tissue on the K_i/K_e ratio, which determines membrane potential. When (K) falls below a certain level, the K_i/K_e ratio begins to decline much more steeply, as is well shown in Fig. 10 of Irvine et al (1961). We have referred previously (p. 17) to the demonstrable effects of severe K depletion on energy production and storage, and on the efficiency of carbohydrate usage and protein synthesis. These fundamental changes are reflected overtly in general malaise and

G

apathy, and more specifically in impaired ability to form a concentrated urine* (Relman and Schwartz, 1955), to secrete acid in the stomach (Carone and Cooke, 1953), to gain flesh after operation (Frost and Smith, 1953), to absorb electrolytes from the bowel (Ariel, 1954), and to maintain normal activity of skeletal muscle (Ferrebee et al, 1941) and the smooth muscle of the bowel (Streeten and Vaughan Williams, 1952). The changes in tissue composition have been reviewed by Darrow (1945); they include low intracellular [K] and [P], with increase in intracellular [Na], while in the E.C.F. there is commonly low [K] and raised [HCO$_3$]. While the pH of plasma and E.C.F. is commonly raised, a fall in intracellular pH has been inferred from CO$_2$ measurements (Gardner et al, 1952), and from the distribution of a weak organic acid, D.M.O. (Irvine et al, 1961). Some of the 'cation gap' within cells may be filled by an increase in basic amino acids (Eckel et al, 1958). Histological evidence of tissue damage was observed by Follis et al (1941) in cardiac muscle and in the kidneys. Cardiac and skeletal muscle (Cohen et al, 1952) show necrosis and disruption of fibres. The observations on heart muscle in K-depleted rats have now been taken to the electron-microscopic level; Molnar et al (1962) regard the damage as mainly cytoplasmic (rather than nuclear) with disorganization of the organelles. The characteristic renal lesion is tubular, a 'clear-cell nephrosis' or 'vacuolar nephropathy' (Conn and Johnson, 1956). The tubular lesions are located in the proximal and collecting tubules (Oliver et al, 1957); and they are associated with changes in the enzymatic pattern of the kidney which can be demonstrated histochemically (Pearse and Macpherson, 1958). Tissue damage similar to that found in animals has also been found in patients dying when severely depleted of potassium (Goodoff and MacBryde, 1944; Perkins et al, 1950; Keye, 1952; Achor and Smith, 1955).

In summary, it may be said from the experimental work that K depletion up to 10 per cent of body-K, an amount comparable to

---

* Because of the importance of the hyperosmotic zone of the renal medulla in the elaboration of a concentrated urine, it is of interest that in K-depleted rats the [Na] in this region of the kidney is abnormally low, and also the concentration of urea (Manitius et al, 1960). The change in [Na] may reflect an impairment of the active process of Na-reabsorption in the ascending limb of Henle's loop.

that lost in diabetic coma or after an uncomplicated surgical operation, produces no definite symptoms, although it does produce
demonstrable biochemical changes. On the other hand, more severe
K depletion causes a widespread biochemical lesion reflected in
general ill-being, in demonstrable dysfunction of many tissues, and
in actual structural changes. The general effects of K depletion have
been reviewed by Welt *et al* (1960), and the renal effects by Relman
and Schwartz (1967).

Clinical Potassium Depletion

CAUSES

In discussing E.C.F. [K], we have already noted a number of
processes which can affect the internal distribution of potassium.
Some of these, such as acidosis, may also increase K excretion, but
most of them do not alter the external balance of potassium. It is
only a net loss of K from the body which leads to true K depletion;
and the causes of this can conveniently be grouped in terms of the
route by which K is lost. Deficient intake of potassium can indeed
produce some degree of K depletion, as has been reported in
anorexia nervosa (Wigley, 1960), for the conservation of K under
conditions of low intake is not so effective as that of sodium; but the
presence of any considerable depletion of K in clinical practice is
always associated with some channel of abnormal loss.

The results of Furman and Beer (1963) indicate that in a 2-hour
period of heat stress amounts of K of the order 5–10 mEq can be lost
in sweat; and Furman (1965) has shown that the K concentration in
sweat can be further increased by exertion undertaken during heat
stress. Whether such losses can result in material K depletion in the
tropics has not been fully explored. In temperate climates, we have
to consider only the alimentary tract and the urine.

ALIMENTARY LOSSES OF K

Intermittent vomiting is not an important cause of K depletion,
probably because the [K] of gastric juice is little higher than that of
plasma, so that even a litre of gastric juice would correspond to only
about a fifth to a tenth of a normal day's intake of K. On the other
hand, pyloric stenosis can lead to considerable K depletion (Burnett

et al, 1950; Davies *et al*, 1956); here the vomiting is associated with semi-starvation, and with wasting of body-tissue which determines a urinary loss of K. Aspiration of gastric and intestinal contents, and copious discharge from fistulae, also produce K depletion, when the intake of K is not augmented. However, these upper alimentary tract losses are less important as a cause of chronic severe K depletion than are losses of K in the stools. There is in the colon a considerable passage of K into the lumen in exchange for Na; whereas the ratio of [Na] to [K] in the secretion of the upper alimentary tract is 20:1, in a formed stool it is only 1:2. When the stools are loose, the Na:K ratio is higher, so that losses of both Na and K are likely, as was found in infantile gastro-enteritis (Darrow, 1946), and also in cholera (Banyajati *et al*, 1960). But whereas Na loss in stools is insignificant when these are 'formed', there can be a very significant loss of K in bulky solid stools; and this has been reported in steatorrhoea (Harrison *et al*, 1943), ulcerative colitis (Lubran and McAllen, 1951), after excessive purgation (Schwartz and Relman, 1953; Litchfield, 1959), after total gastrectomy (Sensenig and Campbell, 1957), and even after repeated enemata (Dunning and Plum, 1956). Potassium depletion is present in the interesting syndrome in which islet-cell tumours of the pancreas are associated with intractable peptic ulceration and watery diarrhoea (Morrison *et al*, 1962). Villous papillomata of the colon and rectum can lead to large faecal losses of potassium (Roy and Ellis, 1959). Sufficient loss of K to produce clinically recognizable depletion has also been reported with exchange resins (Greenman *et al*, 1953); but these are now little used, and those still in use are partly in the potassium cycle.

RENAL LOSSES OF K
These may arise (*a*) as part of a general process of discharge of K from cells; (*b*) as a result of inappropriate excretion of K by normal renal tissue under abnormal hormonal control or other constraint; and (*c*) as a result of renal disease.

(*a*) *'Appropriate' renal behaviour towards K released from cells*. As noted already in discussing K homeostasis within the body (p. 79), potassium is discharged from cells in conditions of Na overload, in acidosis, in dehydration and in excessive protein catabolism. Increased excretion of K has been observed in all these states, and can be regarded as an appropriate response to increased [K] in the E.C.F. Although this is a convenient way of looking at it, we do not wish by doing so to rule out in these states either direct hormonal action on the kidney, or an action of the stimulus directly on renal tubule cells rather than via E.C.F. [K]. Whatever the mechanism, it is worth making some distinction between primary K loss from cells, with secondary renal excretion; and primary K loss in the urine, with consequent depletion of cellular K. de Deuxchaines *et al* (1961) have shown that a low exchangeable potassium is very common in patients, and can only rarely be accounted for by primary losses of K. It can, however, be a necessary part of tissue-wasting, or it may represent 'impairment of cell-metabolism'; the loss of K in both cases is presumably gradual, via the kidneys, and there is little or no retention of administered K, in contrast to true states of K depletion.

(b) *'Inappropriate' excretion of K by structurally normal kidneys, under hormonal or other constraint.* This takes place most notably under the influence of adrenal hormones, whether administered in large doses, or produced in abnormal amounts by adrenal hyperplasia or neoplasm. Potassium depletion has been observed inconstantly in Cushing's syndrome (Willson *et al*, 1940). Bagshawe (1960) suggested that hypokalaemia was much more likely in those patients in whom the appearances of Cushing's syndrome were related to a neoplasm, commonly a pulmonary one; but this view is not supported by the experience of Christy and Laragh (1961). Potassium depletion is the most characteristic aspect of primary aldosteronism; it has even been reported divorced from hypertension, with the interesting suggestion that 'unresponsiveness' of the arterioles to angiotensin might lead to increased formation of angiotensin, with consequent stimulation of aldosterone secretion (Bartter *et al*, 1962). In addition to primary aldosteronism, increased K output in consequence of secondary aldosteronism no doubt contributes to the K depletion which has been observed in cardiac failure (Brenner, 1959; Baum *et al*, 1959), in hepatic oedema (Aikawa *et al*, 1953), in the nephrotic syndrome (Fox and Slobody, 1951), and in water depletion. Severe K depletion has been observed in patients treated with sodium p-aminosalicylate in large doses flavoured with liquorice extract (Cayley, 1950; Strong, 1951). More recently, hypokalaemic palsy has been reported in relation to liquorice preparations used in the treatment of obesity (Gross *et al*, 1966) and—in the form of carbenoxolone—of gastric ulcer (Mohamed *et al*, 1966). As Roussak (1952) points out, the liquorice extract has an action resembling that of adrenal mineralocorticoids (Mulhuysen *et al*, 1950); while the high sodium intake contributes to the E.C.F. alkalosis which has been marked in these patients.

The kidney can also be forced to excrete potassium by agents other than hormones. Both organic mercurials and oral diuretics can produce K depletion, especially in patients on a low intake of sodium. Indeed, the commonest cause of K depletion in the ambulant patient is the prolonged use of diuretics. These increase the amount of Na reaching the distal tubule, where it is available for exchange with cellular K, which is then lost in the urine. As a result of previous diuretic treatment, patients may enter cardiac surgery with a K-deficit (Lockey *et al*, 1966). When diuretics and steroids are given together, as in the treatment of the nephrotic syndrome, considerable losses of K can occur. A systemic acidosis, as we have seen, is associated with loss of K from cells; but in so far as it is attended by an increased excretion of fixed anion not 'covered' by ammonia and hydrion it will also directly augment the excretion of base, which includes potassium. Increased excretion of K has also been observed, however, in alkalosis, whether metabolic (Holliday, 1955) or respiratory (Stanbury and Thomson, 1952); since alkalosis tends to promote the transfer of K from E.C.F. to cells, this effect is probably a direct renal one. The Berliner mechanism whereby a decreased secretion of H is associated with increased secretion of K may well be relevant here. Renal losses of potassium in the absence of renal disease are often traceable to various causes; for example, in diabetic coma the renal loss of K is probably the joint effect of acidosis and glycogen breakdown mobilizing K from cells, and of osmotic diuresis, acidosis and adrenal steroid action increasing the excretion of K by direct action on the kidneys.

(c) *Primary renal disease leading to K loss.* Most patients with renal disease do not lose K abnormally; and in both acute and chronic renal failure, K is commonly retained, or at least there is a tendency to hyperkalaemia. A few patients with chronic renal failure do, however, show inability to conserve K normally; a high proportion of the reported cases have been due to pyelonephritis (Mahler and Stanbury, 1956). Potassium loss associated with urinary infection has been observed to revert to normal with cure of the infection (Jones and Mills, 1964). When renal disease is complicated by hypertensive cardiac failure, and when it involves massive oedema, K loss may take place because of secondary aldosteronism. The diuretic phase of recovery from acute tubular necrosis is at times associated with imperfect conservation of K as well as of Na (Bull *et al*, 1950). Potassium depletion has been reported in the nephropathy associated with the use of out-dated tetracycline (Fulop and Drapkin, 1965). The chronic syndromes of renal tubular dysfunction, such as renal tubular acidosis and the Fanconi syndrome, can also be complicated by K depletion (Milne *et al*, 1952; Stanbury, 1958). Hypercalcaemic nephropathy associated with vitamin-D intoxication (Ferris *et al*, 1961) or hyperparathyroidism (Sanderson, 1967) can lead to potassium wasting. Since K depletion can itself lead to renal tubular dysfunction, the differential diagnosis of patients with combined K depletion and renal damage may be difficult. The occurrence of osteomalacia and of deficient ammonia formation are suggestive of a primary tubular lesion; systemic alkalosis when present favours primary K depletion, but an acidosis does not exclude it, being found both in the tubular syndromes and in primary K depletion. This differentiation is discussed by Stanbury (1958). It has, of course, become further complicated by the realization that diminished renal circulation can cause both hypertension and also stimulation of aldosterone secretion; K depletion in renal ischaemia was reported by Dollery *et al* (1959). Gowenlock and Wrong (1962) report six patients who presented with hypokalaemia and other features of primary aldosteronism, but were found to have renal ischaemia as the probable initiating agent.

CLINICAL PICTURE AND TREATMENT

We have already outlined the effects of hypokalaemia (p. 83), and of experimental potassium depletion of different degrees of severity (p. 86). Confusion has been caused by a failure in many accounts to distinguish between change in plasma concentration of K and change in amount of cellular K; while the distinction of their effects is not rigid, it does serve to explain some observed discrepancies, such as the concurrence of cardiotoxic effects of hyperkalaemia and an overall K deficit (Moore *et al*, 1954). Likewise, failure to differentiate 'moderate' and 'severe' K depletion has clouded opinion on the symptomatology and prognosis, and so on the treatment of K depletion. The amount of K which has actually been lost from the body in any given patient is not easily ascertained, except by balance study or isotope dilution, and even then the estimate is not precise; also, the causes of K depletion, as we have seen, are likely also to cause other electrolyte disturbances. It is for these reasons that we have drawn heavily on experimental studies to support the distinction between 'moderate' and 'severe' K depletion.

Moderate K depletion, with a cumulative negative balance of up to 350 mEq or 10 per cent of total K, is a common condition, occurring whenever the intake of food is interfered with, and often aggravated by increased loss in the stools (gastro-enteritis) or in the urine (diabetic coma). This degree of K depletion probably follows any sizeable surgical operation. The symptoms are not dramatic, unless other factors produce a notable hypokalaemia, in which event a flaccid paralysis may be found. It has often been suggested that quite moderate K depletion can lead to malaise, and this is possible, but has not been proved, nor is it easy to see how it can be. Most of the causes of moderate potassium depletion are self-limiting, or at any rate respond quickly to appropriate treatment. The only general indications for treatment with K salts are the appearance of paralysis with hypokalaemia, and the presence of such complicating factors as might favour continued K loss, e.g. the appearance of ileus during convalescence from an operation. Otherwise, the K deficit will soon be made up when the patient is again eating normally. As Mudge says, potassium 'is best administered by the oral route, preferably in the form of beefsteak'. But in patients who are receiving digitalis, even moderate K depletion carries a potential risk, in view of the serious significance of P.A.T.B., arising from the conjunction of digitalis and K depletion (see p. 84). The moderate loss of K which occurs with the thiazide diuretics is probably the most common precipitant of P.A.T.B.; but it has also been reported with post-operative K depletion, and may indeed limit the use of digitalis after operation (Preshaw and Harvey, 1963). While an acute observer may note jugular pulsation which is rapid and dissociated from the apex-beat, the diagnosis of P.A.T.B. is usually made by the E.C.G. (Oram et al, 1960). When recognized, the condition calls for K administration, intravenously if necessary, and probably also for the intermission of digitalis. Even moderate K depletion may also be specially dangerous in patients with hepatic failure, in whom chloro-thiazide precipitates coma (Sherlock, 1958); Gabuzda (1962) suggests that in K depletion there is an increased renal formation of ammonia and also that the intracellular acidosis of K depletion may favour diffusion of ammonia into cells, giving toxic effects.

Severe potassium depletion is much less common. It is nevertheless important as a cause of puzzling 'attacks' which may be labelled 'neurotic', as a cause of severe and prolonged illness, and ultimately as a cause of death; whereas its recognition can lead to its effective control by specific treatment. While severe potassium depletion arising within a few days is almost always caused by gastro-intestinal disorders with vomiting, diarrhoea or fistulous losses, the chronic states of severe K depletion are quite likely to be of renal origin, though gastro-intestinal causes such as steatorrhoea and abuse of laxatives are also to be reckoned with. The phrase 'of renal origin' must here be interpreted as signifying 'loss by the urinary route', for it includes not only primary renal disease, but also the effects of hydrocortisone and especially aldosterone on K excretion.

The effects of a severe potassium depletion, while serious enough, are somewhat insidious in the sense that a patient may be sustaining renal and myocardial damage with very few symptoms. There may be no more than a general deterioration of health, so indefinite that its onset cannot be dated. Muscle weakness, when present, tends to be episodic, coming on after a carbohydrate meal, which leaves a normal subject indifferent, but will precipitate paresis in a patient with a plasma [K] already low; or else during the night, when there is an increased withdrawal of K from plasma into muscle-cells. Muscular aching may be complained of, also abdominal distension and discomfort. Thirst is a common symptom: it may arise from stimulation of the thirst centre (Fourman and Leeson, 1959) or from neurophypophyseal failure to produce A.D.H. in response to the usual stimuli (Kleeman and Maxwell, 1959); or it may be secondary to polyuria, either that of renal insufficiency, or the A.D.H.-resistant polyuria of K depletion. Aminoaciduria is reported in association with K depletion (Denton *et al*, 1951; Stanbury and Macaulay, 1957; Davidson *et al*, 1960). Albuminuria is common in those patients with primary or secondary renal damage, and the blood urea may be increased, and revert to normal when the K depletion is corrected. Diarrhoea may be present and usually points to laxatives or steatorrhoea as a cause of the K depletion; but diarrhoea with large losses of chloride in the stools has been observed in K depletion as a secondary phenomenon. Oedema has often been observed in patients with K depletion, provided of course that they are not at the same time depleted of Na.

In general, patients with severe K depletion have a plasma [K] below 3.5 mEq/l.; but exceptions to this statement are found in patients with concurrent sodium depletion and oligaemia, and in patients with acidosis. An increase in plasma [HCO_3] to above 31 mEq/l. is also common, together with a fall in [Cl]; but this is of course absent in patients with renal or metabolic acidosis. When the clinical circumstances and plasma findings support a suspicion of severe K depletion, the 24-hour output of K on a low-potassium diet should be determined. At plasma levels of [K] below 3.5 mEq/l. the daily output of K is usually less than 50 mEq. If it is much higher than this, a renal channel of K loss is established, and further investigation must be undertaken to decide whether this is due to renal disease or to the influence of an aldosterone-secreting tumour (Aird *et al*, 1956). On the other hand, a low excretion of K should intensify the search for an alimentary cause of K loss, with careful inquiry into use of laxatives and spontaneous bowel habit, and if necessary a fat-balance. Information can sometimes be obtained by seeing how much K is excreted in the urine after a standard dose of K by mouth (Black, 1953; Kihns, 1954); a low excretion suggests that K is entering tissue cells to replace a deficit. The test is not valid, however, when there is a primary renal loss of K, or on the other hand a generalized renal excretory impairment.

These investigations are, of course, appropriate only to severe K depletion of gradual onset. The problem is somewhat different in patients with alimentary intubation or fulminating gastroenteritis, who can slip into severe K depletion in a few days. Such patients commonly have severe Na depletion as well, which makes the plasma [K] level of little value, and also interferes with urine formation, so that a low output of K does not constitute unequivocal evidence of K depletion. The practical answer seems to lie in awareness of the general risk of K depletion in these circumstances, and a readiness to include K in the fluids used for maintaining fluid balance, especially after the circulation has been restored by correction of the Na deficit. A particular indication of the need to give parenteral K is given by the appearance of paralytic ileus. The concentration of K for intravenous use should not exceed 40 mEq/l.; a solution of this concentration can be given at a rate of a litre in 3 hours. It may be that this recommendation, though in accord with traditional teaching and practice, is in fact unnecessarily conservative, at least when glucose is given at the same time. Kunin et al (1962) found that when K was given at a rate of 20–40 mEq/hour along with $2\frac{1}{2}$–10 per cent glucose, the plasma [K] did not rise, indeed in most patients it fell, sometimes with the production of cardiac arrhythmia. More radically still, Clementsen (1962) gave to two patients amounts of 335 and 375 mEq K intravenously in $5\frac{1}{2}$–$5\frac{3}{4}$ hours, i.e. a rate of over 60 mEq/hour. Almost all the administered K was retained, and there were no toxic effects. These findings in themselves speak for severe K depletion, and this must be well established before massive K loading is undertaken; Clementsen gave his doses in 5 per cent glucose, and also 40–50 units of insulin.

In chronic severe K depletion, parenteral potassium is only very rarely needed, for the control of severe paralysis. Treatment with potassium salts by mouth is given with potassium chloride or bicarbonate in 1 g capsules; with a mixture containing 1 g each of K acetate, citrate and bicarbonate in 8 ml of water (with four doses a day, this supplies 116 mEq of K); or perhaps most conveniently with Mist. Pot. Cit. (N.F.) of which a half-ounce (15 ml) contains 3 g of K citrate, giving 28 mEq of K. In Mist. Pot. Cit. the taste of K salts is masked by ginger; but a similar effect can be attained by effervescent tablets, effervescent granules (Chandler et al, 1961) or the Mist. Pot.

Effervescens (B.P.). Because of the risk of intestinal ulceration, mixtures are preferable to tablets, though there are slow-release preparations of K salts which attempt to forestall this danger. In my view, the alkaline salts of K are preferable, because of their greater palatability (or smaller impalatability), because alkalosis promotes the entry of K into cells, and—more theoretically—because they are appropriate for the correction of the intracellular acidosis which often accompanies severe K depletion. However, it is sometimes necessary to supply chloride as well as K for the complete correction of alkalosis, in which case KCl must be used (Goodwin and Oakley, 1965). For patients with alimentary losses of K, the addition of about 100 mEq of K to the diet will allow the correction of a deficit, once diarrhoea has been controlled; and any excess of K will be excreted by the kidneys. In patients with renal loss of K, the amount of K required has to be assessed for the individual patient. Not only is the amount of daily K loss variable from patient to patient, but an excessive amount of K cannot readily be excreted, and in patients with renal insufficiency there is a risk of K toxicity even with oral dosage. The initial daily requirement of K should be determined from the K loss in the urine on a low-K diet. Thereafter, the patient must be kept under observation, with attention to the possibility of recurrent K depletion and of over-dosage, and checks of the plasma [K] at each visit. Treatment with oral K, once established, has usually to be maintained indefinitely, but these patients are usually willing to co-operate. The striking symptomatic relief obtainable with K salts must not distract attention from curative treatment, when available by such means as weaning from laxatives or the extirpation of an adrenal tumour.

Prophylactic administration of K salts is appropriate for patients on high dosage of cortisone or ACTH, and also for patients undergoing long periods of diuretic treatment, and still more so if they are having digitalis. For these purposes, a supplement of 50–100 mEq/day is adequate.

Hyperkalaemia

An absolute increase in the K content of the body probably does not occur, apart of course from increments in cell-mass during growth or local hypertrophy. Hyperkalaemia has often been interpreted as evidence of K excess, in Addison's disease and in renal failure; but isotope studies indicate that high plasma [K] may exist when the total-body K is apparently depleted (Moore *et al*, 1954). Indeed, there is no recognized syndrome of (K excess + I.C.F. expansion) to correspond with the familiar state of oedema, i.e. (Na excess + E.C.F. expansion). The practical factor which may well prevent the development of such a syndrome, possible in theory, is the high toxicity of any great increase in the concentration of plasma potassium. Drescher *et al* (1958) found that K given to rats was for the most part rapidly excreted; even after death in hyperkalaemia, the total amount of K in the carcass was not appreciably increased. Experimental adrenal insufficiency does indeed lead to some expansion of I.C.F., with K retention, at the expense of E.C.F., which shrinks as Na is lost from the body (Gaudino and Levitt, 1949). Whether a similar situation arises in patients with Addison's disease has not yet been demonstrated, nor are the effects of increased intracellular K known. The important clinical effects of potassium excess are those of hyperkalaemia.

Ingestion of potassium salts causes a transient increase in the plasma [K]; after 10 g of KCl (134 mEq K), the increase is of the order of 2 mEq/l., but it is less with alkaline salts of K. It is possible even in normal subjects to induce paraesthesiae by ingestion of K salts, but frankly toxic levels of [K] are unlikely. Normal animals can of course be killed by intravenous potassium, and the same thing has undoubtedly happened to patients on rare occasions. It has been claimed that dangerous amounts of K may be given in exchange transfusion of the newborn (Campbell, 1955); but it has been shown that the plasma [K] is high in new-born babies, and can even exceed 10 mEq/l. without apparent toxic effects (Widdowson and McCance, 1956). There is evidence, however, that the use of stored blood may be related to cardiac arrest at operation (Le Veen *et al*, 1960). The plasma [K] in stored blood commonly exceeds 23 mEq/l., and blood-loss and cooling are further factors increasing the risk of cardiac arrest. Moreover, Stewart *et al* (1962) draw attention to metabolic acidosis as a factor in surgical cardiac arrest; and this has been shown to be relevant in the dog by Ledingham and Norman (1962).

Spontaneous clinical hyperkalaemia arises when potassium excretion by the kidneys is depressed or absent, and when there is a rapid release of K from cells.* The renal excretion of K may be low in chronic renal failure, but it is not depressed to the same extent as is the G.F.R., and in fact the clearance of K has been observed to exceed that of inulin (Leaf and Camara, 1949; Platt, 1950). It may be for this reason, or because of a low intake of food, that significant hyperkalaemia is exceptional in clinical uraemia, tending to occur only when increased tissue breakdown or administration of potassium increases the amount of K requiring excretion (Fishberg, 1954). The dangers of giving potassium salts to patients with oliguria are not universally appreciated, and the use of potassium citrate as a diuretic and alkalinizing agent in oliguric states must be roundly condemned. In patients with acute renal failure, hyperkalaemia is a notable hazard in the oliguric or anuric phase, and must be avoided by eliminating K from the diet; in practice, this means giving no protein, but giving calories as carbohydrate and possibly as fat. As already mentioned, with the onset of diuresis K may be actively eliminated, and the dietary regime has then to be modified. The hyperkalaemia of Addison's disease and adrenalectomy is partly of renal origin, and administration of aldosterone or DCA increases the output of potassium. The theoretical possibility of spontaneous hypo-aldosteronism without other features of Addison's disease found clinical incarnation in a patient observed in Boston by Hudson et al (1957). This man had spontaneous transient episodes of cardiac arrest, associated with high plasma [K]. These could be induced by K infusion, and reversed by glucose; there was no clinical or chemical evidence of lack of hydrocortisone; and aldosterone was absent from the urine. It is somewhat puzzling that a second patient has been reported with a lack of aldosterone, but with a distinctly different clinical picture, consisting of mild Na depletion with fainting attacks, and with no significant hyperkalaemia (Skanse and Hökfelt, 1958). The problem set by these two patients is considered by Hills (1959) in a thoughtful editorial. Noting that patients maintained on cortisol

---

* An outré example of the conjunction of these two factors follows the bite of a sea-serpent, when widespread muscle necrosis and myoglobinuric nephropathy conspire to give [K] levels toxic to the heart (Reid, 1961).

after adrenalectomy rarely show hyperkalaemia, although they tend to become sodium depleted, he suggests that the patient of Skanse and Hökfelt probably approximates more closely to uncomplicated hypoaldosteronism. The hyperkalaemia in the Boston patient could be due to renal dysfunction, with K retention as a complication. Both patients fulfil the criteria of hypoaldosteronism, given by Hills as '(1) a marked decrease of aldosterone excretion in the urine under circumstances in which it should be present in quantity, and (2) integrity of the glucocorticoid function of the adrenal cortex'. A patient with persistent hyperkalaemia, but with only episodic paralysis, was found by Posner and Jacobs (1964) to have a very low urinary excretion, and also a low secretion-rate, of aldosterone.

The causes of transfer of K from cells into E.C.F. have been reviewed in general terms (p. 80). The clinical states in which such transfers are of importance are increased tissue breakdown associated with trauma and infection; acidosis, as in acute renal failure, diabetic coma and chronic respiratory acidosis; haemolytic crises; and the agonal state with anoxia and general metabolic breakdown. Many of these states also tend to induce renal excretory failure, so that clinical hyperkalaemia is often of mixed origin.

The important clinical effects of hyperkalaemia are its action on the heart, which may cause death at levels of 10 mEq/l. or even lower; and the ascending paralysis, much rarer than the cardio-toxicity, but capable also of causing death from respiratory paralysis.

The cardiac effects of hyperkalaemia are of considerable practical importance as a limiting factor to the rate of K administration by vein, and even by mouth in oliguric patients; as a cause of death in anuria; as a risk of stored-blood transfusion; and as a method of securing prompt but reversible cardiac arrest in surgery. The earliest overt sign of cardiac damage is arrhythmia, followed by a slow idioventricular rhythm, and finally by arrest in diastole, which may be preceded by ventricular fibrillation. There is a somewhat closer correlation between E.C.G. changes and a raised level of plasma [K] than obtains in hypokalaemia; and in the dog successive stages are fairly clear-cut, though the distinction is blurred in man, who also suffers fatal cardiac arrest at levels from 7–13 mEq/l., whereas the dog succumbs to levels of 16–18 mEq/l. The earliest E.C.G. change is peaking or 'tenting' of the T wave; at higher [K] levels this if accentuated, and gaps in sinus rhythm appear. Next, the ventriculas complexes increase in size, and then run together to give a form or biphasic tracing (Fig. 4.2). Final arrest is usually preceded by a slowing

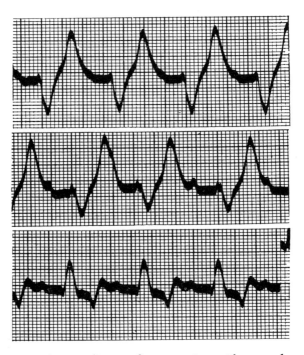

FIG. 4.2. Electrocardiogram from a patient with severe hyperkalaemia, plasma [K] 8.5 mEq/l. Leads I, II, III from above downwards.

of the ventricular beat, but less commonly ventricular fibrillation occurs. Reversal of the earlier changes has often been observed when the plasma [K] falls spontaneously, or is lowered by insulin and glucose. The E.C.G. changes are also modified by digitalis and by intrinsic myocardial disease.

Although direct application of potassium to muscle causes contraction, and even myotonia, in clinical hyperkalaemia the skeletal muscles, if affected at all, are paralysed; though death from cardiac arrest may have taken place without any apparent dysfunction of skeletal muscle. A widespread paralysis of the Landry type, with progressive ascent to involve respiratory muscles, has been reported in renal failure by Finch *et al* (1946); and further cases of hyperkalaemic paralysis were described by Bull *et al* (1953) and by Herman and McDowell (1963). In Addisonian crisis, flaccid quadriplegia associated with hyperkalaemia has been observed (Pollen and Williams, 1960). Numbness and impaired position sense have been observed, suggesting a neuropathy; but the paralysis is most probably due to a block of transmission, not in the end-plate itself, but in the muscle membrane (Adams *et al*, 1953).

Although the principles involved in preventing and treating hyperkalaemia are common to all the conditions in which it occurs, they have been most extensively practised in the management of acute renal failure. The recognition that danger arises from a high concentration of K in the E.C.F. delineates the objectives—to prevent further access of K to the E.C.F., whether from food or from tissue breakdown; to promote elimination of K when possible; to transfer K from E.C.F. to cells; and to give agents which will counteract the cardiac toxicity of [K] in E.C.F.

The diet must be free from potassium. The balance of evidence supports a protein-sparing effect of a high-carbohydrate intake; the difficulty in giving this stems partly from the need to restrict concurrently the intake of water and of protein. Concentrated solutions of glucose cause thrombosis, unless given into the vena cava by catheter; but even this carries some risk of thrombosis and of infection. Parsons and Fore (1963) describe how over 400 g of carbohydrate in the form of liquid glucose can be given orally each day in a limited amount of water. Besides the high carbohydrate diet, other measures to restrict the endogenous supply of K from protein breakdown include the treatment of shock and any definite Na depletion, the control of infection, and the giving of anabolic steroids (McCracken and Parsons, 1958).

In patients without renal failure, e.g. in Addison's disease, the urinary excretion of K should be stimulated with D.C.A. or fludrocortisone. In renal failure, artificial haemodialysis or peritoneal dialysis are applicable. Some K can also be removed via the

H

alimentary tract through the use of exchange resin in the sodium cycle (Evans *et al*, 1953).

Transfer of K from E.C.F. into cells is promoted by giving insulin and glucose, and by the correction of acidosis. Infusion of sodium bicarbonate or lactate is effective in reducing [K], and it may act by lessening the acidosis; but Somlyo (1960) finds that sodium lactate antagonizes not only the effect of hyperkalaemia, but also other myocardial depressants such as quinidine. Other measures to antagonize the cardiac action of hyperkalaemia are digitalization; and the infusion of calcium salts, which have indeed been considered the most effective emergency measure for preventing the dangerous cardiac effects of hyperkalaemia (Chamberlain, 1964). When dialysis is promptly available, it offers a rapid and effective means of correcting hyperkalaemia.

This is simply an outline of the measures available for combating hyperkalaemia. Further details, and also the other important aspects of the management of acute renal failure, are discussed by Merrill (1962) and Schreiner (1967). Levinsky (1966) has summarized the emergency treatment of hyperkalaemia.

CHAPTER V

HYDRION

The above title, an increasingly used package-word for 'hydrogen ion', replaces the phrase 'anions and acid-base balance', used to denote the substance of this chapter in previous editions. This is done deliberately, and in perhaps belated recognition of the advantages to biologists, as well as to chemists, of the Brönsted-Lowry nomenclature of acids and bases. The emphasis is now placed on hydrion itself as the key substance in the 'regulation of the reaction of the body-fluids', to use a term introduced by Robinson (1961) in place of the demoded terms 'acid-base balance' or 'anion-cation balance'; this emphasis is in some ways analogous to the emphasis which we have given in the two preceding chapters to sodium and potassium in the regulation of the volume and tonicity of extracellular and intracellular fluid.

An *acid* is now defined as a molecule or ion which in certain circumstances will give up a proton,* in other words a proton-donor. This definition brings in not only conventional acids such as hydrochloric acid but also the ammonium ion, which can be split into a proton+ammonia, and even water, which splits to give a hydrion + a hydroxyl ion; many anions, such as the chloride ion, are not, on this definition, acidic but are the conjugate bases of a true acid—in the case of chloride, hydrochloric acid. This clear separation between *acidity*, in the sense of donating a proton, and *electrical charge*, which dictates the direction of movement in an electrical field, exemplifies the increased precision which the Brönsted-Lowry terminology makes possible. Conversely, a *base* is defined as a molecule or ion which has a tendency to take up a proton. Ammonia and hydroxyl

* The terms 'proton' and 'hydrion' are used synonymously, and without regard to their hydration in watery solutions to give the hydronium ion, OH_3^+.

ion are strong bases, the addition of a proton yielding ammonium ion and water respectively. Water itself is, in different circumstances, either an acid or a base—as an acid, it loses a proton to yield hydroxyl ion; as a base, it gains a proton to yield a hydrated hydrogen ion ('hydronium'). This ability to lose or to gain a proton earns the epithet 'amphiprotic'. Metallic cations, formerly considered as bases, e.g. in the term 'total base of serum', are neither acids nor bases, since they cannot yield a proton which they do not possess, and they are prevented from taking up a proton by their positive electrical charge. In a reaction such as the neutralization of NaOH by HCl, the Na ion and the Cl ion take no real part, the essence being the transfer of a proton from the hydrochloric acid to form, with the hydroxyl ion of NaOH, water. Another example of the irrelevance of metallic cations to acid-base reactions is the lack of dependence of buffer action on the particular metallic cation used in the salt of a weak acid in the buffer system.

A simple account of the Bronsted-Lowry system from the chemical standpoint is given by Vander Werf (1961). The whole question of the status of hydrion in body-fluid is currently under very active review. An important discussion of the general problems was edited by Nahas (1966). Some account of 'hard' and 'soft' acids and bases (the 'soft' ones being biologically rather toxic, as enzyme poisons) is given by Pearson (1966). Dormandy (1966) develops the relationship between hydrion concentration in the aqueous phase, and oxidation-reduction potential in the non-aqueous phase of the body. These newer concepts have not fully penetrated clinical thinking; but it is with an eye to the future that these key-references are now given.

Whereas the concentration of sodium and potassium in accessible body-fluids is considerable, and can be easily and reproducibly measured by the flame photometer, the concentration of hydrion is vanishingly small, and its accurate measurement is not easy. Not only may loss of carbon dioxide from the sample vitiate the measurement, but error can also arise from the preparation of reference solutions, the type of reference electrode, and the meter used to measure the potential difference between reference solution and sample. The general problems of pH measurement were discussed in a symposium (Woolmer, 1959); for practical purposes, it is desirable to have a convenient and reasonably accurate system of assessing hydrion concentration. Astrup and his colleagues (1960) have now devised apparatus whereby pH can be measured on samples of capillary blood at different partial pressures of carbon dioxide (P_{CO_2}); from this information the nature of the disturbance in hydrion balance can be precisely inferred. As will be seen later, it is necessary to know not only whether hydrion concentration is increased or decreased, but also whether the change has been brought about by metabolic disorder, or by alterations in respiratory or in renal function. The clinical interpretation of [H] and P_{CO_2} in conjunction has been reviewed by Owen et al (1965). Although the Astrup apparatus should now be generally available, it may be worth mentioning that the same inferences can be drawn, though less conveniently and precisely, by combining a measurement of the total CO_2 content of plasma, separated under liquid paraffin, with the measurement of P_{CO_2} by a rebreathing method (Collier, 1956; Campbell and Howell, 1960).

Even granted an acceptable method of determining hydrion concentration, there is discussion as to the best method of expressing the results. A direct statement of hydrion concentration, e.g. $10^{-7.4}$ equiv/l., is clumsy, and for this reason the general practice has been to follow Sørensen's usage of pH, i.e. the negative logarithm, to the base 10, of the actual hydrion concentration (cH or [H+]). This has the disadvantage of expressing increases in concentration as a decrement of the chosen unit. Moreover, a substantial change of cH appears quite small, when expressed in pH units, e.g. a doubling of the hydrion concentration is represented as a fall in pH from 7.4 to 7.1. Robinson (1961) points out how use of the pH unit has established the idea that the reaction of body-fluid is specially closely conserved, whereas in fact the tissues are relatively resistant to change in external [H+]. A doubling of the normal hydrion concentration is compatible with life, which would not be true of either sodium or potassium. As Campbell (1962) shows, the clumsiness of the quantity $10^{-7.4}$ is merely an indication that the wrong unit has been chosen to express concentration. Instead of 'equiv/l.' he advocates the 'millimicroequivalent' (alternatively the nano-equivalent or mµequiv or mμEq per litre). Then $10^{-7.4}$ equiv/l. becomes 40 mμEq/l., and so on. Given estimates of arterial P_{CO_2} (mm Hg) derived from the mixed venous P_{CO_2} determined by the re-breathing method, and of the bicarbonate content (mEq/l.) of the plasma of arterial or arterialized blood, the hydrion concentration H^+ is derived from the formula

$$H^+ = 24 \frac{P_{CO_2}}{HCO_3^-} \text{ m}\mu\text{Eq/l.}^\star$$

This relationship is shown graphically in Fig. 5.1 (p. 111)

Hydrion Homeostasis

Hydrion differs from sodium and potassium, and resembles water, in that during its transit through the body from ingestion to excretion it does not maintain its identity, but is constantly disappearing into or emerging from the complex of chemical reactions which constitutes energy metabolism. This prevents the rigid application of the concept of 'balance' to the hydrion household; just as water balance includes the somewhat nebulous moiety 'water of oxidation' (p. 19), so the intake of actual hydrion is negligible compared with the hydrion which will be generated in the oxidation of food and tissue. The combustion of carbohydrate and fat produces carbon dioxide, which dissolves to give carbonic acid; the combustion of protein likewise produces carbon dioxide, but in addition other acids are formed, including 'mineral' acids such as sulphuric and phosphoric acid and also organic acids, including the keto-acids. As Elkinton (1962) points out in a useful review, the massive production of CO_2 in metabolism does not involve a *net* excretion of hydrion by the lungs; when retention of CO_2 occurs in respiratory disease, there is a higher ratio of $H.HCO_3/B.HCO_3$, and so an increased hydrion concentration in plasma, but the total hydrion being produced in

---

$\star$ To select values such that the arithmetic at least is tolerable, a (normal) P_{CO_2} of 40 mmHg and plasma bicarbonate of 24 mEq/l. can be entered in the

formula to give $H^+ = \dfrac{24 \times 40}{24} = 40$ mμEq/l.; this corresponds to a pH of 7.4.

metabolism is not increased. There are three main sources* of metabolic hydrion:

(1) Incomplete oxidation of carbohydrate and fat, to organic acids.

(2) Oxidation of sulphur-containing amino acids to give sulphuric acid (Hunt, 1956).

(3) Oxidation and hydrolysis of phosphoprotein residues (Relman et al, 1961).

This non-volatile hydrion, amounting to some 70 mEq per diem, cannot be eliminated by the lungs, but is dealt with by urinary excretion. Although the urine is normally acid, the free hydrion is negligible by comparison with that excreted in combination with buffer as 'titratable acid' and with ammonia as ammonium ion $(H^+ + NH_3 \rightarrow NH_4^+)$.

The general picture, then, is of a metabolic production of hydrion in two main forms—in part 'potential hydrion', or CO_2, which can be eliminated by the lungs; but also the non-volatile hydrion of organic acids, and of sulphuric and phosphoric acid, which can only be excreted by the kidneys (in the form of ammonium ion and titratable acidity). This is the approach in terms of balance, but its value is limited by the variety of unknown components on the 'positive' side of the balance. Hydrion regulation can also be looked at from the point of view of the factors regulating the hydrion concentration in plasma. Recalling that [H] is proportional to the ratio $P_{CO_2}/[HCO_3]$, we are once again concerned with the lungs and the kidneys: in that the level of P_{CO_2} is determined by the drive of the respiratory centre and the efficiency of the lungs; while the renal conservation of bicarbonate is complementary to the renal excretion of acid (and indeed depends on it to some extent, as the filtered bicarbonate joins with secreted hydrion in the proximal tubule to form $H_2CO_3 \rightarrow H_2O + CO_2$, both of which are readily reabsorbed).

The degree to which the hydrion concentration of arterial plasma is allowed to vary is greater than would be inferred from a casual glance at the normal range of pH from 7.44 to 7.36; as explained above, a truer picture is given by the range of actual concentration,

---

* In addition to these three sources, generation of hydrion from phospholipide can assume importance on certain diets (Ardaillou and Richet, 1966).

from 36 to 44 mμEq/l.—a 20 per cent variation.* This represents a degree of biological control similar to that for serum [K], whose normal range is 3.9–5.0 mEq/l. When sudden changes occur in the production of hydrion within the body, the effect on plasma H is minimized by the action of buffers both in blood and tissue, and by exchange of hydrion with the metallic cation of bone (Bergstrom, 1956). These actions mostly take place rapidly, and the respiratory response to change in plasma [H$^+$]—or, more accurately, to [H] in cerebral extracellular fluid (Pappenheimer, 1965)—is also rapid, giving a prompt appropriate change in P$_{CO_2}$. The renal adaptation is slower, and it takes some days for maximum change in hydrion output in the urine (or renal conservation of bicarbonate) to occur. Also, the full extent of buffering by bone salt is a long-term affair, although it can then reach notable proportions (Lemann et al, 1966).

More detailed accounts of the short-term and long-term regulation of hydrion have been given by Pitts (1963), Relman (1964), Robertson (1965), and Elkinton et al (1967). As we have seen, the permitted range of hydrion concentration in extracellular fluid is fairly wide; but Elkinton points out that it is also precarious, in that the total daily turnover of metabolic hydrogen (70 mEq) is 'more than half the total amount of hydrogen normally present in all the buffers of the body, and one-tenth the maximal hydrogen storage capacity of these buffers'. The ratio of turnover to body-content is perhaps some measure of the vulnerability of homeostasis; in comparison with the value of 50 per cent for hydrion the corresponding values are about 4 per cent for water, 5 per cent for sodium, and 2.5 per cent for potassium. Although the percentile variation permitted in [H$^+$] is considerable, the absolute variation is minute, the change being measured in mμEq. Attention has (quite reasonably) been concentrated on the changes in [H] in the extracellular phase, where it can be routinely measured. Intracellular [H] is no doubt more variable still—and that within the same cell, in which there will be local sites of metabolic generation of hydrion. Even if the idea of 'intracellular

* It is perhaps an unfortunate coincidence that the digits 36 and 44 are common to the two modes of expression—actually, pH 7.44 corresponds to [H] of 36 mμEq/l.; and is thus representing a lower quantity than pH 7.36, which corresponds to 44 mμEq/l.

[H]' is a statistical concept, methods are now available for quantitating it, and some of the factors which regulate it are being studied Adler *et al*, 1965). Most estimates of cellular pH have been around 7.0, but a recent careful study, using glass micro-electrodes implanted intracellularly in the muscle, suggests a much lower figure—around 6.0 (Carter *et al*, 1967).

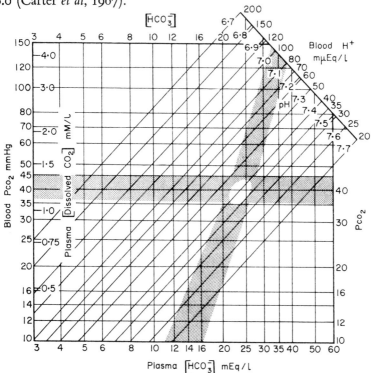

FIG. 5.1. Logarithmic plot of blood P_{CO_2} and plasma [HCO_3], to give blood [H]; a graphic expression of the Henderson-Hasselbalch equation. The normal ranges for P_{CO_2} and [HCO_3] are shaded, except for the clear ovoid at the intersection, which indicates normal resting arterial conditions. I am indebted to Dr E.J.M. Campbell and to the Editor of the *Lancet* for permission to reproduce the figure.

'Acidosis': Hydrion-excess

This may be defined as an excess of actual or potential hydrion within the body. The term is not synonymous with acidaemia, which means an excessive concentration of hydrion in the plasma; for example, an increase in respiration may conserve a normal hydrion concentration in plasma even when excessive hydrion is being produced in metabolism. The state of acidosis without acidaemia has been referred to as 'compensated acidosis'; this is not a stable situation, and tends to break down into 'uncompensated acidosis' if the metabolic cause of hydrion excess persists. In a similar fashion, retention of CO_2 (potential hydrion) in early respiratory failure can be 'compensated' by increased renal retention of bicarbonate; but with continued or increasing respiratory failure, acidaemia is added to acidosis. There are many causes of acidosis, but they can be classified under the general headings:

Metabolic acidosis—excessive production of hydrion.

Renal acidosis—defective renal elimination of hydrion.

Respiratory acidosis—defective respiratory elimination of potential hydrion.

Metabolic acidosis. As we have seen, the metabolic production of actual and potential hydrion is a normal phenomenon. It is accentuated by a diet rich in sulphur and phosphorus (i.e. in protein); by a diet which allows the incomplete oxidation of fat (a ketogenic diet); and by forced exercise, which leads to incomplete combustion of carbohydrate, to lactic acid rather than fully to CO_2 and water. This normal production of hydrion, and its normal occasional excesses, are counterbalanced by continuous or increased activity of the lungs and kidneys. Essentially similar processes can be accentuated or prolonged in disease to a degree which outstrips the ability of the normal defences to cope with them. For example, the excessive protein breakdown in fever, starvation, or dehydration can lead to excessive hydrion production and to acidosis. The breakdown of effective carbohydrate metabolism in uncontrolled diabetes lays an extra charge on protein and on fat, leading to excessive protein breakdown, and to incomplete combustion of fat, with ketosis.

Acceleration of normally occurring processes of hydrion formation is only one of the possible mechanisms of metabolic acidosis. Another quite direct mechanism is the administration of substances which are either themselves acids (i.e. hydrion-donors), or which form acids in the course of their breakdown (e.g. methanol, broken down to formic acid). The loss from the body of alkaline fluids, such as pancreatic juice and faecal fluid, represents a subtraction of hydroxyl ion: this is the equivalent of an addition of hydrion, in an aqueous medium, since $H^+ + OH^- \rightleftharpoons H_2O$; so that unbalanced hydrion will be formed from water whose hydroxyl ion is removed from the system. Even the addition of sodium chloride to the body leads to acidosis, although no hydrion is being supplied from without; the mechanism here seems to be a dilution of the bicarbonate in body-fluid, so that the equilibrium $H_2CO_3 \rightleftharpoons H^+ + HCO_3^-$ is shifted to the right, giving increased actual hydrion formation from dissolved CO_2, which is itself only potential hydrion. This phenomenon, described by Shires and Holman (1948) as 'dilution acidosis', perhaps represents acidaemia rather than true acidosis as defined above; it has some practical importance in limiting the speed with which sodium chloride can be given intravenously. On the basis of their observation that acidosis is produced by infusion of glucose or mannitol, as well as of saline, Asano *et al* (1966) support the view that the acidosis induced by saline infusion is a consequence of dilution per se, and not an effect of the chloride ion. A similar conclusion would arise from the animal studies of Winters *et al* (1964), who used in dogs mannitol and urea, as well as hypertonic NaCl.

Another form of metabolic acidosis which has been fairly recently recognized is 'lactic acidosis' (Huckabee, 1961); there is an increased plasma lactate, and the patients are critically ill. This condition has now been reported in severe circulatory insufficiency (Mackenzie *et al*, 1964; Neaverson, 1966)—and also following extra-corporeal circulation; apart from tissue hypoxia, lactic acidosis has been observed in hepatic glycogenosis, and has been experimentally produced by guanidine intoxication (Minot *et al*, 1934). The diguanide oral hypoglycaemic agents inhibit aerobic glycolysis; and lactic acidaemia has been reported as a cause of acidosis, without ketosis, in diabetic patients (Daughaday *et al*, 1962). The possibility of lactic acidosis has clear relevance to the use of sodium lactate in the treatment of acidosis (Schwartz and Waters, 1962).

Metabolic acidosis, however induced, tends to raise plasma [H]; and this probably always happens to some extent, in spite of efficient compensating processes. These include an increased respiration, which lowers P_{CO_2} in conformity with the reduced bicarbonate of plasma; storage of hydrion in the buffer-systems of blood and of tissues, a rapid if somewhat limited mechanism; and the slower adaptation of the kidneys to excrete more hydrion (Pitts, 1963). It should be noted that increased respiration and the action of buffers are efficient in limiting acidaemia, but do not directly dispose of metabolically produced hydrion; the long-term correction of metabolic acidosis depends on the changes in renal function. These various adjustments are apparent in a lowering of plasma P_{CO_2} and bicarbonate, some rise in [H], and the formation of a urine of high [H] and ammonium content.

Renal acidosis. The kidneys are concerned in the disposal of metabolically produced actual hydrion, and only minimally in the disposal of potential hydrion, which is dealt with by the lungs. To some extent, therefore, renal acidosis is a subdivision of 'metabolic acidosis'; but it seems worth while to preserve the distinction between excessive production of metabolic hydrion, and its defective renal elimination. As indicated by Wrong (1962), the renal elimination of hydrion can be analysed into three components:

(1) hydrion expended in neutralizing filtered bicarbonate
(2) hydrion excreted as titratable acid
(3) hydrion excreted as ammonium.

These are summed up in the well-known expression for renal excretion of hydrion $-H^+ = T.A. + NH_4 - HCO_3$, in which the positive terms represent components (2) and (3), while the negative term expresses the extent to which component (1) is failing to occur.

Impairment of each of these processes of hydrion excretion has been observed in patients with renal disease.

(1) *Bicarbonate wastage.* Schwartz et al (1959) showed that some patients with renal failure and acidosis could have their acidosis corrected by alkalies; as they redeveloped acidosis, renal excretion of bicarbonate accounted for a substantial proportion of their retention of hydrion. This was not a constant finding, and bicarbonate wastage is probably only an exceptional cause of renal acidosis, though other examples of it have been recorded.

(2) *Impaired excretion of titratable acid.* The quantity of hydrion excreted in this form depends both on the concentration of hydrion which can be achieved by secretion into the tubular fluid, and also on the amount of buffer available. In the syndrome of renal tubular acidosis, the ability to concentrate hydrion in the urine (i.e. to produce a urine of low pH) is grossly impaired. Even in renal tubular acidosis, a degree of glomerular insufficiency is frequent, and this will aggravate the situation by restricting the availability of buffer; there will then be a still lower excretion of titratable acid than would be possible at the same urinary pH if the buffer content were normal. The second of these factors also operates in the acidosis of generalized renal failure, when a low glomerular filtration limits the available buffer; but the ability to concentrate hydrion is not impaired in glomerular failure, as indicated by the low urinary pH which can be attained. The satisfactory state of the tubular part of the process of acidification in chronic renal failure has been further demonstrated by Elkinton (1962); when corrected for loss of nephrons, i.e. the glomerular component, the kidneys were maintaining the bicarbonate level of plasma at a level higher than the predicted, an index of effective response to the acidosis imposed by loss of glomerular function. There is, however, some evidence in patients with pyelonephritis (Kleeman et al, 1960) and hydronephrosis (Berlyne, 1961) of a defect in urinary acidification out of proportion to the degree of general renal impairment. Hellman et al (1965) found evidence that parathormone in excess impaired the ability of the kidney to concentrate [H] in tubular urine.

(3) *Impaired excretion of ammonium.* Even though the tubules in chronic renal failure are remarkably competent in many ways (Platt, 1952), in the matter of ammonia formation they are limited by the substrate brought to them; and it is an old observation, confirmed and extended by Wrong and Davies (1959) that the excretion of ammonium in generalized renal disease is much impaired. On the other hand, patients with renal tubular acidosis had often no impairment of ammonium excretion, and some were even excreting sufficient hydrion as ammonium to compensate for their failure to concentrate hydrion. This compensation of course is lost when the progression of renal damage impairs glomerular

function, with which ammonium excretion is closely correlated. In addition to general renal failure, and specific tubular syndromes, whose importance as causes of renal acidosis is implied in the above account, a failure of renal excretion of hydrion may arise when the kidneys themselves are quite healthy, but have an inappropriate pattern of function imposed on them. In Addison's disease, ammonia formation can be inadequate, and acidosis can occur. Diuretic agents which act by inhibiting carbonic anhydrase interfere with tubular secretion of hydrion: this was an important effect with acetazoleamide, but the newer thiazide drugs have very little effect on carbonic anhydrase even in effective diuretic dosage, and their use does not lead to systemic acidosis. In patients with a uretero-sigmoid anastomosis, there is commonly an ascending infection, and pyelonephritis is a recognized cause of renal acidosis; but the situation is aggravated by some reabsorption of acid from urine stagnant in the bowel (Lowe et al, 1959).

Respiratory acidosis. This is most commonly seen as a result of airway obstruction, such as may complicate chronic bronchitis. By comparison with faulty ventilation, disturbances of distribution and of diffusion are unimportant in causing CO_2 retention, though they are of course potent causes of anoxia. The much greater diffusibility of CO_2 than of O_2 implies that in a diffusion defect fatal anoxia would occur before any significant degree of CO_2 retention; and in disturbances of distribution the efficiently ventilated moiety of alveoli can blow off additional CO_2, but they cannot of course add significantly to the already high O_2 saturation of the blood leaving them. A detailed account of the respiratory mechanisms underlying CO_2 retention is given by Campbell (1963). Besides emphysema, CO_2 retention may be due to an insensitive respiratory centre from disease or drugs; to weakness of the respiratory muscles, and inadequate artificial respiration; and to air-way obstruction. For the reasons just outlined, CO_2 retention can never be simply assumed to be present on the basis of proven respiratory disease and anoxia, but must be demonstrated by estimation of the P_{CO_2} in mixed venous or arterial blood.

If a solution of constant bicarbonate concentration is exposed *in vitro* to different partial pressures of CO_2, the hydrion concentration will vary directly with the P_{CO_2}; or in terms of pH, there will be a fall in pH of 0.3 unit if the P_{CO_2} is doubled, and conversely the pH will increase by 0.3 unit if the P_{CO_2} is halved. *In vivo*, the effect of adding a corresponding amount of CO_2 is much less, because there are buffers in plasma other than bicarbonate, and also because the plasma is not in isolation. The retained CO_2 diffuses into the tissues, with a lesser rise in P_{CO_2} than the same increase of CO_2 would produce *in vitro*; and the bicarbonate concentration no longer remains constant, but increases partly as a result of increased renal tubular reabsorption of bicarbonate (Pitts, 1963). Even in the nephrectomized dog, however, the extracellular buffer mechanisms account for only some 3 per cent of the compensation for acidosis induced by breathing 20 per cent CO_2; the role of tissue exchange of Na and K for H^+ is preponderant (Giebisch, Berger and Pitts, 1955). The increase in bicarbonate is not adequate to compensate entirely for the effect of the raised P_{CO_2} in raising hydrion concentration, so the plasma shows a rise in [H], in spite of the increase in buffer which is mainly accounted for by increased bicarbonate. As Robinson (1961) and others have pointed out, this increase in bicarbonate buffer is potentially confusing, and indeed misleading when only bicarbonate is measured; either the P_{CO_2} or the pH must also be estimated. In view of the increase in buffer, Robinson has suggested 'acidaemia' rather than 'acidosis' as the term to describe the effect of CO_2 retention; but this suffers from the disadvantage of focusing attention on the plasma, whereas the most important change may be an increase in the $[H^+]$ of tissue cells, associated with the increased P_{CO_2} of the body generally. One evidence of increased $[H^+]$ in tissue cells is the increased renal-tubular secretion of hydrion, which is the probable basis of increased bicarbonate reabsorption and the formation of an acid urine. Carter, Seldin and Teng (1959) found that respiratory acidosis in rats was associated with a persistent increase in the excretion of potassium, suggesting that cell cation was being 'displaced' by hydrion, as is well known to occur in metabolically induced acidosis. Carter *et al* (1959) also showed that the renal adaptation to respiratory acidosis differed from that to metabolic acidosis, in that there was no increase in renal glutaminase or carbonic anhydrase.

In an important series of studies, W. B. Schwartz and his colleagues have observed the effect, on plasma [H], of increasing the carbon dioxide content of inspired air in normal men; and have compared these results with the situation in chronic respiratory acidosis. In the acute experiments, Brackett, Cohen and Schwartz (1965) found that for each mm. rise in P_{CO_2} there was an increase of 0.77 nanomoles (nM or mμM) of [H] per litre. When P_{CO_2} was increased from 40 to 90 mm, [H] rose from 40 to 80 nM/l., whereas bicarbonate rose only from 25 to 28 mM/l. This contrast is well illustrated in their Fig. 5. In chronic hypercapnia, however, the same group (van Ypersele de Strihou et al, 1966) found much higher levels of [HCO_3], implying lower [H] at any given level of P_{CO_2}. The 'carbon dioxide titration curve' is therefore much less steep in the chronic situation (in which renal compensation has had time to occur). Sapir et al (1967) have further shown that hypoxia without hypercapnia does not alter the slope of the carbon dioxide titration curve, so presumably the explanation of the changed slope in chronic respiratory disease does not lie in hypoxia. Cohen and Schwartz (1966) have reviewed the situation in pulmonary insufficiency.

Clinical aspects of acidosis. In discussing the types of acidosis, and the mechanisms by which they are produced, we have referred at intervals to the clinical states associated with acidosis; but it may be useful to summarize them now (Table 5.1) in a list which is not exhaustive, but is aimed at illustrating mechanisms. While information of this nature may suggest that a patient may have acidosis of a given type, a more precise characterization can only be based on the estimation of at least two of the components of the Henderson-Hasselbalch equation,* or the equivalent non-logarithmic formulation given on p. 108.

The demonstration in this way of a raised blood [H^+]—or a low pH—confirms the presence of acidosis. If the P_{CO_2} and [HCO_3^-] are increased, the acidosis is respiratory in origin; in both metabolic and renal acidosis the P_{CO_2} and bicarbonate concentrations are low. In metabolic acidosis, the urine has a high [H^+] (low pH), and a high

$$* \, pH = 6.1 + \log \frac{[HCO_3]}{[H_2CO_3]}$$

output of ammonium. In renal acidosis, there is either a low ammonium excretion relative to the pH of the urine, or the pH itself may be high relative to the degree of systemic acidosis. When there is

TABLE 5.1

Clinical causes of different types of acidosis

Metabolic acidosis

Excess hydrion production in metabolism
    from protein: catabolic response to trauma and fever
    from fat: ketosis of starvation and diabetes
    from carbohydrate: lactic acidosis in anoxic and terminal states
    from phospholipide: high intake of egg yolk.
Increased intake of acid or 'potential acid'
    Diets high in protein and fat. Ammonium chloride, methanol, aspirin.
Loss of base
    Pancreatic juice, fluid stools.

Dilution acidosis

Renal acidosis

Impaired formation of ammonia. Generalized renal failure.
Defective hydrion secretion. Renal tubular acidosis, pyelonephritis and hydronephrosis.
Extrarenal causes of defective urinary acidification. Carbonic-anhydrase inhibitors. Addison's disease. Uretero-sigmoidostomy.

Respiratory acidosis

Ventilatory failure from air-way obstruction
    insensitive respiratory centre
    paresis of respiratory muscles.
Carbon-dioxide poisoning.

doubt as to whether an acidosis is renal or metabolic, and the acidosis itself is not too severe, the response to a standard load of ammonium chloride (Wrong, 1962) may help both in establishing the presence of a renal acidosis, and also in deciding whether it is a part of general renal impairment, or due to specific tubular dysfunction. The 'hydrogen ion clearance index' of Elkinton *et al* (1960) is a useful way of relating hydrion excretion (UV$_{H^+}$, expressed as

I

$meq/min/1.73$ m^2) to the degree of systemic acidosis, which is assessed as the reciprocal of plasma CO_2 content in mM/litre (an assessment which is not applicable, of course, to respiratory acidosis). The index, evaluated from the formula $H.C.I. = \dfrac{UV_{H^+}}{1/[CO_2]plasma}$, has a normal range of 1.4–3.4: patients with metabolic acidosis have a normal or high index, while patients with renal acidosis have indices falling well below the normal range (Elkinton, 1962).

The clinical effects of acidosis are not easy to distinguish from those either of the primary condition or of associated disturbances of body-fluid such as uraemia or sodium depletion in renal and metabolic acidosis, and hypercapnia in respiratory acidosis. Patients with respiratory acidosis are often aware of respiratory discomfort, due to the causal condition rather than to the acidosis itself; patients with metabolic and renal acidosis often do not complain of dyspnoea, even though they are grossly hyperventilating (Kussmaul breathing). Irregular jactitation of the limbs is seen in many patients with acidosis, not all of whom are uraemic; it is sometimes relieved by hypertonic sodium bicarbonate, and this differentiates it from hypocalcaemic tetany, which would be aggravated by partial correction of acidosis, and is also more prolonged and painful, whereas the jactitation associated with acidosis is brief and apparently without distress. Experimental acidosis can make animals comatose, and pH values below 7.25 are associated with mental disturbances and coma in man. In respiratory acidosis, the situation is confused by anoxia and hypercapnia; but the relief of anoxia may diminish ventilation further, and in such patients the aggravation of mental disturbance must be related either to hypercapnia or to the acidosis. Scribner (1958) has made the critical observation that patients with respiratory acidosis can be brought round from coma by perfusing the stomach with sodium bicarbonate, a measure which will diminish acidosis but not hypercapnia. There are suggestions that correction of acidosis may relieve bronchospasm (Lancet, 1965), and lessen the likelihood of cardiac arrest (Stewart et al, 1965).

As with many other disorders of body-fluid, the most vital part of the treatment of acidosis is an attack on its cause. In metabolic acidosis, the metabolic disorder must be corrected if possible, e.g. by insulin in diabetic ketosis; sources of acid in the diet or regime are to be sought and eliminated, and losses of alkaline fluid checked. Renal acidosis can usually only be palliated, but defective urinary acidification from extrarenal causes, e.g. in potassium depletion, can be treated specifically. In respiratory acidosis the main treatment is that of the primary disorder. However, it may be necessary to treat the acidosis directly, as an emergency measure, to give time for more radical treatment to be effective; this can be done by infusing sodium bicarbonate or sodium lactate. Sodium lactate, in M/6 solution, has been most generally used; but hypertonic (molar) lactate is advisable when there is hyponatraemia, and bicarbonate must be used instead of lactate when there is any question of lactic acidosis. In the longer-term palliation of renal acidosis, the Shohl mixture of sodium citrate and citric acid for oral use has proved its value, though sometimes potassium citrate should partly or wholly replace sodium citrate (Milne et al, 1952). To meet the case when acidosis should be corrected without adding to the body either sodium or potassium salts, Hurst et al (1963) studied the value of anion exchange resins given by mouth. These could take up chloride, sulphate and phosphate in the alimentary tract, in exchange for hydroxyl, bicarbonate and carbonate ions, each of which could neutralize hydrion retained in the body, to give readily excreted water or carbonic acid. Studies in normal subjects suggested that resins would exercise some such effect and would be more effective than calcium salts or aluminium hydroxide. More recently, organic buffer (THAM) has been used to correct acidosis without the addition of metallic cation to the body (Bleich and Schwartz, 1966).

'Alkalosis': Hydrion Deficit

The normal course of metabolism tends towards an excess of hydrion, to be disposed of by the kidneys, and less directly by the lungs. As we have seen, the commoner metabolic disturbances tend to increase hydrion production; and impaired renal and pulmonary function, by restricting the elimination of hydrion, will likewise tend to produce acidosis. It is not therefore too surprising to find that alkalosis is seldom a spontaneous state, but arises from the imposition of alkali loads on the body, or from the excessive activity of normal lungs, which as it were, dispose of hydrion beyond the call of duty, in response to an emotional or even a mechanical drive. These two mechanisms correspond to 'metabolic' and 'respiratory' alkalosis; while one can conceive of renal mechanisms which would lead, for example, to an excessive elimination of hydrion,* a spontaneous 'renal alkalosis' has never been clearly shown. However, Wrong (1962) draws attention to the difficulties which renal disease may bring in the elimination of imposed loads of alkali: this is not limited to glomerular failure, with its diminished filtration of base (potential hydroxyl ion), but may be present in tubular syndromes, in which Pak Poy and Wrong (1960) have found a low urinary P_{CO_2}. This implies that for any given urinary pH bicarbonate excretion will be less than in normal urine; the excess of bicarbonate so reabsorbed will neutralize hydrion within the body, giving a tendency to alkalosis. While patients with renal disease are vulnerable to alkali dosage, and may even at times show changes in function such as could lead to a spontaneous 'renal alkalosis', the recognized categories of alkalosis are the metabolic and the respiratory.

Metabolic alkalosis. It has been established by Sanderson and his colleagues (Van Goidsenhoven *et al*, 1954) that patients without renal or metabolic disease can tolerate very large doses of sodium bicarbonate, up to 116 mM (140 g) per diem for 3 weeks. There was indeed an alkalaemia, with raised bicarbonate, and a relatively much smaller rise in pH; but this was not progressive, and renal function was not impaired. Sodium was retained, and the E.C.F. expanded, but these changes, once established, were likewise not progressive. The need to eliminate hydroxyl ion rather than hydrion must be a rare event in the life of carnivorous and omnivorous animals, but it is general in the herbivora, as witness the classical observation of Claude Bernard on the alkaline urine of rabbits, which became acid only when starvation forced them to feed on their own flesh. In species which feed irregularly, and so at times hugely, the sudden call

---

* One such mechanism is the avid reabsorption of bicarbonate, seen in K depletion, and probably based on a raised intracellular hydrion concentration (Roberts *et al*, 1956).

for massive peptic secretion can leave the body awash in an alkaline tide. Coulson *et al* (1950) describe the notable case of the alligator, which can eat a quarter of its weight at a meal, after which the blood pH rises to over 8, while the [Cl] falls from 100 to 40 mEq/l. In spite of the relative rarity of the stimulus in nature, the response to loading with alkali is extremely efficient, as shown by Pitts and his colleagues (see Pitts (1963) for a detailed review). The *renal response* consists in a massive excretion of bicarbonate, a mechanism whose appropriateness was stressed by Gamble (1954); huge amounts of potential hydroxyl ion are eliminated in this way without the pH of the urine having to exceed 7.8 (Gamble's chart 24). Although metallic cations such as sodium are not in themselves bases, loading with alkali in effect means loading the body with a metallic cation combined with an anion which is disposed of in metabolism or in expiration; and the response to alkali loading demands the excretion of metallic cation along with a readily available anion, and not an anion like chloride, whose supply is limited. The mechanism of real quantitative importance is the use of bicarbonate in this way: the daily respiratory elimination of carbon dioxide is of the order of 15,000 mM, so that a 1 per cent decrease in this would retain in the body 150 mM of CO_2, which in body-fluid could potentially give 150 mEq of bicarbonate available for excretion with cation in the urine, and 150 mEq of hydrion to neutralize the excess of alkali.★ A possible subsidiary mechanism for increasing cation excretion in the urine without expenditure of chloride was suggested by Cooke *et al* (1954), who showed that in rats given large amounts of $NaHCO_3$ there was little loss of Cl in the urine; the eliminated sodium was associated not only with bicarbonate, but also with considerable amounts of citrate and other tricarboxylic acids. Evans *et al* (1957) have since shown that this response is much less striking in man, and is practically limited to citrate. It may even be that the increased excretion of organic acid is not an adaptation, but a necessary consequence of the alkalinity

★ The smallness of the percentage change in ventilation called for to cope with any reasonable load of alkali makes me willing to condone those impercipient people, like myself, who have never been convinced of their ability to detect clinically the 'hypopnoea of alkalosis'; in my experience, this observation follows, and does not precede, a biochemical revelation.

of the urine; many non-ionized organic acids are more diffusible than their corresponding anions, so that they could enter the tubular urine by diffusion, and then be 'trapped' there in a medium more alkaline than intracellular fluid, which would increase their ionization. The process of non-ionic diffusion has been reviewed by Milne *et al* (1958); it has important implications in the excretion of acidic and alkaline drugs.

The *respiratory response* of underventilation, which we have already noted as a contributor of bicarbonate for the renal elimination of base, is also effective in correcting alkalaemia. Addition of base to the body, or abstraction of hydrion from the body, leads to an increase in plasma bicarbonate; decreased elimination of CO_2 ensures that this increase in bicarbonate is partly or wholly matched by an increase in dissolved CO_2, so limiting or preventing the fall in [H], as determined by the ratio $[HCO_3]/[BHCO_3]$.

Cannon *et al* (1965) have described under the heading *contraction alkalosis* a phenomenon which appears to represent the converse of the 'dilution acidosis' discussed on p. 113. When vigorous diuresis is induced, there is loss of Na and Cl, but not of HCO_3; so that in effect the same amount of HCO_3 is distributed in a smaller volume of E.C.F. The consequent increase in $[HCO_3]$ is not attended by a corresponding rise in P_{CO_2}; so there will be a fall in the ratio of $P_{CO_2}/[HCO_3]$, and consequently a fall in [H].

Respiratory alkalosis. The critical event here is excessive respiratory elimination of carbon dioxide, with a lowering of the arterial P_{CO_2}, and of the carbon dioxide content of the body. The term 'hyperventilation' is commonly used to describe this state of affairs, but it is not always strictly accurate; when the P_{O_2} of the inspired air is reduced, a level of ventilation which is barely adequate for oxygenation may be excessive in terms of CO_2 elimination. Does this constitute hyperventilation? The most adequately studied form of respiratory alkalosis is the form induced by voluntary hyperventilation, in which any anoxic complication is lacking. Reduction of P_{CO_2} (and so of $H.HCO_3$), without primary change in $B.HCO_3$, produces a fall in [H]. To control the extent of this, both extra-renal and renal mechanisms are evoked. In the nephrectomized dog, Giebisch *et al* (1955) showed that the extrarenal mechanisms which limit a fall in extracellular [H] included transfer of cation from E.C.F. to I.C.F., and access to the E.C.F. of Cl from red cells, and lactate from the muscles. The general effect of these ionic transfers is to limit the fall in [H]. Given that [H] depends on $H_2CO_3/BHCO_3$, and that H_2CO_3 is primarily lowered, these transfers induce a cognate fall in $BHCO_3$, some of the 'B' escaping into cells, while the $-HCO_3$ is replaced by Cl and lactate. This redistribution of bicarbonate represents a rapid but temporary means of mitigating the alkalinizing effect of a lowered P_{CO_2}; it is quickly supplemented by an enhanced renal excretion of bicarbonate in an alkaline urine (Stanbury and Thomson, 1952). This depression of renal reabsorption of bicarbonate is closely correlated with the fall in P_{CO_2}* (Pitts, 1963) and may well depend on a fall in intracellular [H] (Maren et al, 1961).

CLINICAL ASPECTS OF ALKALOSIS

When hydrion is rapidly lost from the body, either by spontaneous vomiting or by gastric suction. an acute *metabolic alkalosis* develops. This state of acute hydrion depletion responds quite well to the administration of NaCl, or of NH_4Cl; renal function is good, and if chloride is supplied the accompanying cation is of little import. When vomiting or suction are repeated or prolonged, the situation is complicated by the loss, in addition to hydrion and chloride, of significant amounts of metallic cation, both sodium and potassium; renal function is impaired, and simple replacement of chloride is inadequate to correct the alkalosis. The administration of ammonium chloride in chronic alkalosis is inadequate, since it aggravates sodium and potassium depletion, and can also lead to ammonium poisoning. Depending on the chronicity of their vomiting, and on their intake of sodium salts, patients with pyloric stenosis have been shown to suffer in varying degree from depletion of chloride, of sodium, and of potassium (Davies et al, 1956). While alkalosis in the E.C.F. is common to these states, acute alkalosis can be corrected by NaCl,

* Rector et al (1960) have shown that bicarbonate is reabsorbed in the tubules by at least two processes—one directly related to plasma P_{CO_2}, unaffected by inhibitors of carbonic anhydrase, and probably in the proximal tubule; the other independent of P_{CO_2}, sensitive to inhibition of carbonic anhydrase, and located distally.

whereas in slowly developing alkalosis K depletion is present, and must be corrected before the alkalosis will respond fully to treatment (Roberts *et al*, 1954).

Depletion of chloride, with or without some accompanying depletion of Na and K, is probably a much commoner cause of alkalosis than is the massive and prolonged ingestion of soluble alkali in patients with peptic ulcer. Gastric aspiration, with concomitant replacement of KCl and NaCl, but not of HCl, was studied by Needle *et al* (1964); for complete correction of the consequent alkalosis, replacement of Cl was needed. Alkali ingestion is a clear-cut situation in comparison with the alkalosis of chloride loss; and the first descriptions of clinical alkalosis were in patients taking large doses of sodium salts (Hardt and Rivers, 1923; Cooke, 1932; Cope, 1936). Even before the high tolerance to alkalies had been shown experimentally, it had been questioned whether some additional factor to alkali ingestion, such as renal insufficiency, was also required for the development of clinical alkalosis (Hardt and Rivers, 1923). A high intake of calcium can apparently aggravate the effects of alkali ingestion, a concept embodied in the term 'milk-alkali syndrome' (Burnett *et al*, 1948). Since calciferol poisoning by itself can produce renal calcification, thirst and nausea, mental disturbances, and renal failure, the precise part played by the alkalies in the milk-alkali syndrome is in some doubt, especially as calcium salts were often included in alkali mixtures (Cope, 1936). Cope gives anorexia and nausea as early symptoms, and apathy, mental disturbance and coma as later symptoms of alkalosis; and notes that typical symptoms have been seen when potassium citrate was given for pyelitis, suggesting that calcium intoxication is not a necessary mechanism of the syndrome.

Tetany occurs in patients with alkalosis secondary to vomiting, but is unusual in patients who owe their tetany solely to the ingestion of alkalies. This difference is no doubt related to the normal, or even raised serum-calcium in the latter group; whereas in the former the lowered plasma [H] not only depresses the ionized fraction of calcium, but may also have a direct action on neuro-muscular irritability. The degree of uraemia is equally variable in different patients with metabolic alkalosis, and the only constant biochemical features are those of the alkalosis itself—raised plasma pH and bicarbonate, and also P_{CO_2}. In the patients who have ingested alkali, the urine is usually alkaline, but in patients with electrolyte depletion, the urine may be acid. This 'paradoxical aciduria' may be due to enhanced bicarbonate reabsorption secondary to raised P_{CO_2}, or—more probably—to complicating K depletion which leads to enhanced renal tubular secretion of hydrion.

The commonest clinical cause of *respiratory alkalosis* is the semi-voluntary hyperventilation which is one form of response to anxiety. Increased ventilation is a physiological response to low environmental P_{O_2}, and some of the symptoms of mountain sickness are related to hypocapnia. Analeptics, fever, encephalitis and hypothalamic tumours can all cause hyperventilation. Respiratory alkalosis is a frequent accompaniment of long-term management of poliomyelitis in a respirator (Thomson, 1957). In salicylate intoxication, the primary effect on acid-base balance is a central stimulation of respiration, leading to respiratory alkalosis; this is shortly complicated by K depletion, which may then outlast the alkalosis itself (Robin *et al*, 1959). Hypocapnia has also been described after intracranial haemorrhage, and attributed to stimulation of the respiratory centre by increased C.S.F. [H] derived from glycolysis of the added blood (Froman and Crampton Smith, 1966). During recovery from pulmonary embolism, hypocapnia is observed.

The symptoms associated with episodic hyperventilation are extremely varied; interesting groups of symptoms have been described by Lewis (1954) and by Singer (1958). Commonly, the patient feels that he cannot get breath, and struggles against this feeling to such purpose that he is soon tingling in every limb, and cramped in spasms of tetany. It is worth asking patients with 'odd feelings' and 'attacks' whether their symptoms are preceded by any sensation of choking or breathlessness. If the patient can be persuaded—and this is not always so—to overbreathe in the clinic, the reproduction of his symptoms may pave the way to an assurance of their innocent character. Alternatively, the cutting short of an attack by re-breathing into a paper bag—or, for those who like complication, a Douglas bag—may equally be made the basis of reassurance. However, recognition of hyperventilation in association with other symptoms does not mean that the syndrome can be easily cured; for the symptoms apparently secondary to hyperventilation may be those of an anxiety state, and not truly dependent on the hyperventilation at all. This point is well made by Saltzman *et al* (1963), who showed that forced ventilation for an hour in normal subjects did not reproduce any of the 'effects' complained of by patients after a few minutes' over-breathing. Similarly, patients on long-term artificial ventilation can be alkalotic without any dramatic symptoms; they have, therefore, to be monitored at reasonable intervals, especially as they may demand a level of ventilation in excess of their true needs (Thomson, 1957). The essential biochemical pattern of respiratory alkalosis is a fall in blood [H] and in P_{CO_2}, but in contrast to metabolic alkalosis the plasma bicarbonate is diminished. The urine is commonly alkaline, and contains bicarbonate, but these findings are not invariable, especially if the situation is complicated by K depletion.

It may be apparent from this account of the clinical aspects of alkalosis that neither metabolic nor respiratory alkalosis are very common effects of disease; and that when they do occur, as in patients with vomiting or undergoing artificial ventilation, they are very likely to be complicated by other disturbances. Whereas a direct attack on acidosis by giving alkaline solutions is sometimes justified, I am doubtful if a direct attack on alkalosis by giving acids (or potential acids such as ammonium chloride) is ever called for. Management consists in removing or adjusting the predisposing causes, and in attending to other disturbances of body-fluid.

Relation to Other Disorders of Body-fluid

From time to time in this brief account we have found it necessary to introduce changes in Na, K and Cl balance as complications, or even as explanations, of changes in acid-base balance. The new emphasis on hydrion has perhaps made it easier to give a straightforward description of primary acid-base disturbance; but the time has now come to do fuller justice to the influence of changes in other ions on the acid-base balance. There are numerous minor interactions of this sort; for example, the production of an acid urine is enhanced by a low-sodium diet, or one which supplies poorly reabsorbable anions such as sulphate. There is, however, a more clearly defined relationship between potassium depletion and acid-base balance; and some recent work suggests that chloride may have a rather specific role in the correction of alkalosis. These two topics, which are perhaps only examples of similar relationships, may now be considered.

Hypokalaemic alkalosis. Although this term has been criticized on linguistic grounds, and perhaps deserves more serious criticism in relation to its accuracy, it is nevertheless difficult to devise a substitute. The situation which it describes is a combination of low [K] and raised bicarbonate in the serum, which is also of low hydrion concentration (raised pH). It is generally regarded as a manifestation of potassium depletion: but it is worth noting that many patients with K depletion do not exhibit hypokalaemic alkalosis: and that the same biochemical picture is seen in patients with primary alkalosis (in which K is excreted in the urine, and also enters cells from the E.C.F.) and in patients who have been intensively treated with diuretics, especially mercurial diuretics, which are alkalinizing in their effect (Schwartz and Wallace, 1951). In both these latter situations, there may indeed be a degree of potassium depletion, but it is not the primary event. However, there is no doubt that a primary experimental K depletion can lead to hypokalaemic alkalosis, provided there is an adequate intake of sodium (Black and Milne, 1952).

Losses of sodium from the body, e.g. in watery diarrhoea, tend to be associated with acidosis; and it has never been clear why depletion of another metallic cation, i.e. potassium, should often be associated with alkalosis. A convincing explanation of this anomaly was given by Cooke *et al* (1952); having observed that the K lost from cells in states of K depletion was only partially replaced by Na, they suggested that there might be an increase of hydrion in the cells, i.e. an intracellular acidosis. If the intracellular excess of hydrion is greater than the extracellular deficit, the overall situation will be an acidosis. This explanation is sometimes summarized as 'a shift of hydrion from E.C.F. to I.C.F.'; but this cannot be an exact description, as there is insufficient hydrion in E.C.F. to account, if transferred, for the required degree of intracellular acidosis. Moreover, any change in hydrion content of I.C.F. must be heavily buffered by phosphate and protein. The combination of extracellular alkalosis and a greater intracellular acidosis is, however, supported not only by the original balance results of Cooke *et al* in rats, but also by the balance results in human experimental K depletion (Black and Milne, 1952), and in patients recovering from pyloric stenosis (Davies *et al*, 1956). There are, of course, criticisms of the comparison of the balance of $(Na+K)$ and of (Cl) as a basis for inferences about hydrion; but the concept of an intracellular acidosis is more directly supported by the observation of Irvine *et al* (1961) that the intracellular pH of normal rat muscle is 6.92, while the muscle of K-depleted rats has a pH of only 6.69 (the corresponding [H] values, of course, are 120 mμEq/l. and 202 mμEq/l., which perhaps gives a more striking view of the increase in [H], while equally making it plain that an increase of this order would make little difference to total cation concentration, which is measured not in mμEq/l., but in mEq/l.).*

An alkalosis with hypokalaemia sometimes complicates the hypercapnia of chronic respiratory failure—a confusing situation, because there is usually a respiratory acidosis. The conjunction of hypokalaemia, raised bicarbonate, and alkalosis (*high* pH) was first observed by Refsum (1961), and again by Cochran (1963). In a fuller analysis, Robin (1963) suggests that alkalosis and hypercapnia in respiratory disease may arise in several ways. Therapy with diuretics may lead to potassium depletion, giving at least an extracellular alkalosis. When P_{CO_2} is acutely lowered by artificial ventilation, renal excretion of bicarbonate may lag behind. Finally, there is the possibility that chloride depletion, the consequence of long-standing respiratory acidosis, may delay the fall in bicarbonate concentration which would normally take place when P_{CO_2} is brought down. This last possibility, of a specific role of chloride in relation to acid-base balance, warrants fuller study.

Chloride and acid-base balance. The critical observations here were those of Schwartz and his colleagues (1961). When dogs made hypercapnic by breathing 12 per cent CO_2 were allowed to recover, on a

* On the other hand, in careful studies Miller *et al* (1963) were able to find only small and inconstant changes in cell pH when rat diaphragm was acutely depleted of K in a bath; the relevance of these observations to gradually developing K depletion *in vivo* is doubtful.

low chloride diet, the bicarbonate fell to some extent, but did not fall to normal levels until chloride was supplied. They suggested that the active reabsorption of sodium in the proximal tubule generated a potential difference, which was lessened by concurrent reabsorption of chloride; when Cl was not adequately available for this purpose, the secretion of hydrion, and also of K, was enhanced. Later the same group showed that full recovery from hypokalaemic alkalosis was also dependent on a supply of chloride (Atkins and Schwartz, 1962); and that substitution for chloride of a poorly reabsorbed anion such as nitrate would also lead to excessive secretion of hydrion, with a consequent alkalosis and raised level of bicarbonate (Gulyassy et al, 1962). The clinical relevance of these experimental observations has been demonstrated by Aber et al (1962). They studied six patients with hypokalaemic alkalosis (two with upper bowel obstruction, two with diarrhoea, and two with Cushing's syndrome); in all of them repletion of K did not suffice to correct the alkalosis, whereas the additional provision of chloride effected full recovery from the alkalosis. Further evidence of the critical role of chloride in correcting alkalosis in certain patients has come from studies by de Graeff et al (1964), Kassirer et al (1965), and Luke and Levitin (1967).

Although in this chapter the Brönsted-Lowry terminology, and the substitution in many places of [H] for pH, has been accepted, we have not used either 'whole-blood buffer base' (Singer and Hastings, 1948) or 'standard bicarbonate' (Astrup et al, 1960). This is a deliberate omission, in the belief that these systems tend to confuse independent disturbances with adaptations to existing disturbances; and that they add to the complexity of the subject rather than alleviating it. Moreover, the emphasis on in vitro behaviour of a whole-blood sample neglects the importance of tissue buffering of hydrion disturbances. This is the position adopted by Schwartz and Relman (1963); it does not detract from the great practical value of the Astrup apparatus in the measurement of [H].

CHAPTER VI

AN APPROACH TO
TREATMENT

It has always seemed to me that the help which books and papers can give in the treatment of patients is severely limited. In dealing with disorders of body-fluid, it is possible to describe pure syndromes in some detail; and this has been attempted in the preceding chapters. Such a description is, however, two stages away from practical treatment. Firstly, the pure syndromes, like Platonic universals, scarcely deign to show themselves in this workaday world. Secondly, even an accurate theoretical diagnosis has to be obtained in what amounts to a different way for each patient, and the consequent treatment must be again fitted to the patient. The process by which theory is transmuted into practice eludes description: but something can perhaps be said of the points in clinical examination and chemical investigation which are most relevant to body-fluid disorders; and an outline of available therapeutic methods can also be given.

Most books on this subject include several chapters on the electrolyte disturbances most commonly found in a number of diseases. This leads to much repetition of what has already been said in describing the general syndromes of electrolyte disorder; and it also implies a rather one-sided presentation of many subjects which are more naturally dealt with in general text-books of medicine and surgery. More important, it encourages the fallacy of thinking that because a patient is suffering from X, he will also have Y and Z; whereas he need not have either. While the assessment of electrolyte disturbance can be assisted by knowledge of the primary disease, this information is of less importance, in the present context, than a general knowledge of the causes, effects and management of electrolyte distortions. I have therefore limited this type of information to a simple list (Table 6.1) of the most usual electrolyte disturbances found in association with a number of common diseases and syndromes.

In this table, D represents a deficit, and E an excess of a substance denoted by the subscript, e.g. E_K represents 'potassium excess', and D_{H_2O} 'water depletion'. 'Ac' and 'Alk' are used for acidosis and alkalosis. In some cases (E.C.F.) and (I.C.F.) follow the other symbols to indicate the localization of a limited disturbance. Where a convenient reference is available, it is given in the last column. Diseases and syndromes in alphabetical order. Obviously any list of this type is incomplete both as a whole and in its separate parts; and the division into 'predominant' and 'subsidiary' disturbances is somewhat arbitrary.

It is opportune, however, to notice here a rather general pattern of abnormality in nitrogen and electrolyte metabolism which accompanies trauma, surgical operation, and probably also severe 'medical' disorders. Foreshadowed by the earlier work of Selye on the 'alarm reaction', and of Peters and Cuthbertson on the accelerated protein catabolism after burns and trauma, the 'metabolic response to surgery' was described at length by Moore and Ball (1952). Little has been added to their account on the descriptive level, except that we now know many more contexts in which this response occurs. The observed changes are oliguria for 24–48 hours, increased excretion of nitrogen and potassium, and retention of Na and Cl. The oliguria is based on reduced renal blood-flow to some extent, but to a much greater extent on increased secretion of A.D.H., in response to pain, anaesthesia and morphine. The pattern of electrolyte excretion suggests the action of aldosterone, and there is some evidence of increased aldosterone activity following surgery (Llaurado and Woodruff, 1957). A possible stimulus to this would be decreased volume of body-fluid, and Flear and Clarke (1955) suggested that the metabolic response to injury could be prevented by adequate transfusion. However, Timoner et al (1959) found no difference in the metabolic response to gastric surgery when extra blood was transfused.

A 'permissive' rather than an essential role has been ascribed to the adrenal cortex, based on observations that the 'metabolic response'

TABLE 6.1

	Disturbance		
Disease or Syndrome	Predominant	Subsidiary	References
Addison's disease	DNa, H_2O: EK	EUrea: Ac.	Loeb (1941-42)
Coma	DH_2O	DNa, K: Ac.	Marriott (1947)
Congestive heart failure	ENa, H_2O	DKEUrea: Ac.	Moyer and Fuchs (1960)
Cushing's syndrome and high cortisone dosage	ENa DK	Alk. (E.C.F.)	Christy and Laragh (1961)
Diabetic ketosis	DNa, H_2O: Ac.	DK	Nabarro et al (1952)
Diarrhoea			
Acute (gastroenteritis)	DNa H_2O	DK: Ac.	Darrow (1946)
Chronic (sprue, colitis)	DK	DNa	Schwartz and Relman (1953)
Haemorrhage, shock	ENa, H_2O	DK	Moore and Ball (1952)
Heat effects	DH_2O, Na		Ladell et al (1944); Leithead and Lind (1964)
Hepatic insufficiency	ENa H_2O	DK	Summerskill (1960)
Hyperventilation (functional or in encephalitis)	Alk.	DNa, K	Stanbury and Thomson (1952)
Intestinal obstruction	DNa, K, H_2O	Ac.	Wangensteen (1942)
'Nephrotic syndrome'	ENa H_2O	DK	Fox and Slobody (1951)
Periodic paralysis	DK (E.C.F.)		Danowski et al (1948); Zierler and Andres (1957)
Post-operative state	ENa, H_2O DK		Moore and Ball (1952)
Pulmonary failure	Ac.	ENa, H_2O DK	Platts and Greaves (1957)
Pyloric stenosis			
Acute onset	DCl, Alk.	DNa	Davies et al (1956)
Chronic with alkali medication	DNa, K, Cl EUrea	Alk. (E.C.F.): Ac.(I.C.F.)	Davies et al (1956)
Renal failure			
Acute-oliguric phase	ENa, K, H_2O, urea		Bull et al (1950)
Acute-polyuric phase	DNa, K		
Chronic	EUrea Ac.	ENa or DNa: EK or DK	Fishberg (1954)
Tubular syndromes	Ac: DNa or K or H_2O		Stanbury (1958)
Undernutrition	ENa, H_2O	DK	McCance (1953)

still occurs after adrenalectomy in patients kept on a fixed supplement of cortisone. This would suggest that variation in the response of tissues to injury is not entirely fixed by variation in the amount of hormones reaching them, but is partly determined by the previous state of the tissues themselves. Previous trauma and general malnutrition greatly diminish the metabolic response to later injury; and apart from this the degree of response is partly conditioned by the amount of injured tissue.

With relation to fluid therapy, the chief lesson to be learned from studies on the electrolyte changes after injury is that while blood-replacement must be adequate, patients who have sustained tissue damage are unable to excrete water, Na and Cl normally, and should not therefore be loaded with these substances. The loss of K which is also part of the metabolic response to trauma is usually quite small, and assumes importance only as a contributory factor when other causes of K depletion are also present; only in the presence of such complicating factors is active treatment with potassium salts required.

History and Examination

Much of the information needed to assess fluid balance comes from a thorough general history and examination. The special points to keep in mind are whether there has been any interference with intake or any abnormal loss of electrolytes and water; and whether the patient has any symptoms or signs which could easily be explained by recognized syndromes of fluid depletion or excess.

GENERAL IMPRESSIONS

Patients with disturbances of body-fluid are often gravely ill, but need not be so. Even in ambulant patients, oedema may be obvious, as may muscle weakness or mental confusion; the voice may be altered by lack of saliva. Severe sodium depletion produces the appearance known as clinical dehydration, in which a skin fold is lax and the underlying tissue flabby and scanty; this appearance is exaggerated by wasting, and obscured by obesity. The eyes may be partly occluded by facial oedema; or unnaturally staring in severe sodium depletion.

K

Patients in bed can show similar changes on superficial examination. They may also already be festooned with tell-tale tubes when first seen by a physician; and these tubes may be a cause of fluid imbalance in an attempt to cure it. Posture in bed can speak of apathy, of muscle-weakness, of bone-pain. The breathing may suggest pulmonary oedema, or rarely respiratory paresis, with 'fish-mouth breathing'. The hyperpnoea of severe acidosis has to be distinguished from voluntary hyperventilation (largely by its persistence) and from dyspnoea; the shallow breathing of alkalosis is (to me at least) often visible only by hind-sight.

ALIMENTARY TRACT

Deficient intake is caused by anorexia, by apathy and weakness, and of course by coma. General weakness may bear more hardly on the intake of water than of food and minerals, for in a busy ward patients may be assisted at meal-times, but not so regularly encouraged to drink at other times. Vomiting and watery diarrhoea are obvious ways of losing fluid, as are intestinal suction and discharge from fistulae; the loss of electrolyte, and especially of potassium, in bulky formed stools is more easily overlooked.

Thirst has been stressed as a distinctive evidence of water depletion; but many patients with depletion of sodium or of potassium also complain of it. The tongue is dry and coated and the saliva scanty in sodium depletion; indentation of the tongue margins by the teeth may be apparent in sodium excess. Abdominal distension with absent bowel-sounds can be caused by potassium depletion.

URINARY SYSTEM

This comes second only to the alimentary tract as a frequent channel of electrolyte loss; as a cause of electrolyte retention, it shares dubious honours with the heart and liver. In the history, points to be noted are previous renal disease, past or present dysuria, and changes in urine volume. Patients can be surprisingly unaware of what measurement shows to be a striking oliguria; polyuria may be little noted during the day, but is obvious to the patient as increasing nocturia. Physical examination may help by showing a large bladder or a tender kidney, but quite often tangible evidence of renal disease comes first from examination of the urine, or even from the finding of a raised blood urea.

CIRCULATION

Primary disorders of the circulatory system are important causes of sodium excess, and to a less degree of K depletion. Moderate sodium depletion may show itself as postural fainting, with hypotension; while severe sodium depletion is one of the commoner causes of peripheral circulatory failure, with hypotension even in recumbency, cold extremities and collapsed thready veins. Cardiac irregularity and electrocardiographic changes are important effects of K depletion and excess. Abnormal cardiographic patterns are also found in other electrolyte disturbances (Goodwin, 1958).

NERVOUS SYSTEM AND MUSCLES

Coma is a cause of water depletion, and when prolonged of electrolyte depletion as well. It may also be a consequence of acidosis, of hypernatraemia, of severe K depletion—or, perhaps most commonly, of a combination of electrolyte disturbances. Weakness of muscles, which may extend to respiratory involvement, may be related either to low or to high plasma [K]; with severe K depletion, there may be actual necrosis of muscle cells, including the myocardium. The converse symptom of tetany may be spontaneous, or need stimulation of the motor nerves to elicit it.

RESPIRATORY SYSTEM

As a cause of electrolyte disturbance, pulmonary failure is most directly important in relation to respiratory acidosis and alkalosis, and as the primary cause of the oedema of cor pulmonale, though this is of course directly mediated by cardiac and renal dysfunction. Sodium excess, especially when conjoined with hypertension or mitral stenosis, may be first manifest clinically as exertional or nocturnal dyspnoea.

MISCELLANEA

Renal failure, so commonly associated with and aggravated by disorders of body-fluid, may be first revealed by bone-pain, or by the proximal muscle weakness associated with azotaemic osteo-dystrophy (Stanbury, 1962). Otherwise occult renal failure may also appear in the tiredness, pallor and dyspnoea of an anaemia which is shown by investigation to be normocytic. Functional hyperventilation is the mechanism by which some of the bizarre symptom-complexes of the psychoneuroses are produced. The ocular tension may be perceptibly low in severe sodium depletion, but other clinical evidence of this is usually more reliable. Cramps are common in acute water overload, but also occur in many otherwise normal people. Rapid gains and losses in weight are usually due to change in body-fluid. In the management of patients with anuria, or under-going repeated dialysis, regular weighing is of great value in the control of fluid-balance. In severe sodium depletion, there may be pyrexia although the extremities are cold (dehydration fever). Although the impact of water depletion on the circulation is in general less than that of sodium depletion, fever has been observed under extreme conditions of water-loss (Shaker, 1966).

Carpenter et al (1965), in a useful analysis of the clinical features of patients with cholera, noted that the blood-pressure and pulse-rate could be normal even when there was considerable Na depletion; and Yahr and Krakauer (1965) also observed normal B.P. and pulse in patients whose fluid-deficit, as assessed from the central venous pressure, had reached 25 per cent of the initial value. The quality of the pulse, and the state of the neck veins, were found helpful by Carpenter et al; and also changes in the voice, described thus: 'ab-normalities of phonation, varying from a feeble hoarse whisper to complete loss of voice, was present in all patients of the series, but these abnormalities rapidly disappeared' [with rehydration].

Awareness of the frequency of electrolyte disturbances and their multi-potentiality as a cause of symptoms is only a small part of clinical medicine; but the relative ease and success with which some of them can be treated give it added practical importance. Before proceeding to treatment, however, some biochemical investigations should be made, as a corollary to the clinical judgment of the situation. The most important biochemical tests are those which establish the nature of the lesion causing electrolyte disturbance, when this is not clinically apparent. For example, in renal acidosis the detection of faulty acidification of the urine points the way to an alkalinizing regime of treatment; and in respiratory acidosis the investigation of pulmonary function and the blood gases is more relevant than the level of plasma $[HCO_3]$ and $[H]$ at any given moment. However, a text-book of medical investigation cannot readily be fitted into a chapter of a short book on body-fluid, so I shall only mention here some points on the significance and limitations of the measurements which are likely to be carried out in any disturbance of body-fluid. This limits the field to readily accessible fluids and methods, i.e. the estimation of $[Na]$, $[K]$, $[H]$, $[Cl]$, $[HCO_3]$ and a few non-electrolytes in plasma, urine and occasionally in vomitus, fluid stools and fistulous discharges.

Laboratory Investigations

PLASMA
Samples of blood for analysis can usually be obtained from an antecubital vein, though on one or two occasions in a collapsed patient I have obtained blood from the femoral vein. About 20 ml of blood should be taken, as the high haematocrit of sodium depletion may make the yield of plasma smaller than usual. The specimen should be transferred to a heparin tube containing an inch of liquid paraffin, and centrifuged within 30 minutes of sampling; dry tubes with liquid paraffin can also be used, with centrifuging to yield serum. Haemolysis invalidates estimation of the plasma $[K]$, because of the high $[K]$ of erythrocytes; syringes and needles used must therefore be dry, and the blood must not be roughly handled in transfer from syringe to centrifuge tube. Well-tried methods for Na, K, Cl and HCO_3 are described in standard manuals of clinical chemistry, and with flame photometry the results of these estimations can be available within an hour of sampling. The estimation of $[H]$ has been greatly eased by the Astrup apparatus, and replication is made more practical by the small sample needed.

Thompson and Sherwood Jones (1965) have noted disquieting errors in the results for serum electrolytes, as analysed and reported in district laboratories. The interpretation, of even accurate results, has certain limitations, the main ones being that they represent concentration and not total amount, and that they refer only to one phase of body-fluid at one particular time. Nevertheless, they often serve to call attention to disturbances which revaluation of the clinical picture may then establish; and when carried out serially, they give useful information on the progress and complications of treatment. Even when biochemical results are not available, effective treatment need not be totally despaired of; in cholera patients, it was found that the intravenous fluid-requirement could be clinically evaluated with considerable accuracy. The validity of the amounts chosen for replacement was checked in retrospect by specific gravity results on serum, which had not been available at the time of the emergency assessment (Carpenter *et al*, 1965).

The plasma *sodium* lies between 137 and 148 mEq/l. in 80 per cent of normal people (Wootton and King, 1953). The significance of plasma [Na] is stated or implied in Chapter III, but the main points affecting its practical interpretation may be conveniently summarized here. Since [Na] represents 95 per cent of the cation concentration of E.C.F., it is a convenient index of the osmolality of E.C.F., and by inference of the osmolality of body-fluid generally.* The implied assumption that plasma [Na] represents E.C.F. [Na] is less valid when the protein or lipid content of plasma is grossly abnormal. Apart from this, a raised plasma [Na] implies hyper-osmolality of E.C.F., and a low plasma [Na] hypo-osmolality of E.C.F.; such a change need not imply a primary disturbance of sodium balance, but can equally well be produced by change in water or potassium balance. For example, in water intoxication the plasma [Na] is as low as, if not lower than, the plasma [Na] in severe sodium depletion. As Edelman *et al* (1958) point out, hyponatraemia may reflect either (a) primary sodium deficit, (b) primary potassium deficit, (c) primary water excess, or (d) combinations of these. The further transition from E.C.F. osmolality to I.C.F. osmolality is possibly invalid when the energy metabolism of the cells is impaired by disease. For these

---

* The [Na] is not, of course, as precise an index of plasma osmolality as is direct measurement of osmolality itself; when facilities are available for rapid freezing-point determination of osmolality, they avoid the occasional confusion which may arise from high concentrations of glucose or urea (see p. 30, footnote).

reasons, a low plasma [Na] is useful confirmatory evidence of sodium depletion in a patient who is losing saline fluid and who has the general symptoms of Na depletion; but it should never be the only indication for giving sodium salts. A raised plasma [Na] is much more commonly the result of water depletion than of a primary Na excess, which indeed is often accompanied by normal or even low [Na] in oedematous states. Apart from administration of hypertonic saline solutions, the main recognized cause of raised [Na] without water deficit is primary aldosteronism—which is perhaps another way of saying that raised [Na] from sodium excess, as opposed to water depletion, is rather uncommon.

The plasma *potassium* lies between 3.9 and 5.0 mEq/l. in 80 per cent of normal people. As an index of potassium depletion, low plasma [K] has its limitations, reviewed in Chapter IV, of which the effects of change in E.C.F. volume and of acidosis and alkalosis are the most important. These limitations are less critical in chronic states of K depletion, because there are fewer complicating factors of this type; and a low value of plasma [K] is usually found in chronic depletion, whether of gastro-intestinal or of renal origin. With the exceptions of periodic paralysis and high loading with dextrose, a plasma [K] below 3.0 mEq/l. is good evidence of K depletion; but a [K] in the normal range does not exclude K depletion. The relationship between plasma [K] and K balance was reviewed by Scribner and Burnell (1956). A raised plasma [K] in a non-haemolysed sample* is important evidence of potassium excess, and, by dialysis or other means, calls for urgent treatment to prevent cardio-toxicity. Such treatment may sometimes consist in the control of an acidosis, which is raising the plasma [K], rather than in a direct approach to K balance. Raised plasma [K] is one of the few biochemical findings which it is justifiable to treat in its own right, once errors in collecting or analysing the sample have been excluded.

The plasma *hydrion* normally ranges from 36 to 44 nano-equivalents (mμEq) per litre. The corresponding pH range is 7.44 to 7.36.

---

* An artefact which rarely arises, but should be kept in mind, is seen in patients with greatly increased platelets, which—like erythrocytes—have a high K content; this can occasionally give a misleading rise in the apparent serum [K] (Hartmann and Mellinkoff, 1955).

An estimate of [H], either directly by electrometric apparatus, or inferentially from P_{CO_2} and [BHCO$_3$], is necessary for the appraisal of acid-base disorders (see Chapter V). An increase in plasma [H] directly demonstrates acidaemia, but in almost all circumstances acidosis can be inferred. Also, a fall in plasma [H] demonstrates alkalaemia; while this usually implies alkalosis, there is the situation of K depletion, in which alkalaemia and acidosis co-exist. To decide whether an acid-base disturbance is of respiratory or of metabolic origin, the [H] alone is not enough. Rapid changes in [H] are possibly more suggestive of a respiratory than of a metabolic disturbance; but the ultimate distinction between them has to be based on the general clinical situation, and on other biochemical information, including the plasma-bicarbonate and P_{CO_2}.

The plasma *chloride* is normally between 101 and 106 mEq/l. As the main anion of E.C.F., chloride concentration participates in those general changes which are more precisely delineated by the plasma [Na]; and the main interest of [Cl] lies in those instances where its behaviour deviates from that of [Na]. A low [Cl] in relation to [Na] suggests either a metabolic alkalosis or a respiratory acidosis; and conversely a raised [Cl] suggests metabolic acidosis or respiratory alkalosis. The relationship is not very precise, however, because of the relative infrequency of chloride retention in relation to acidosis. While it is important in renal acidosis, and especially in the acidosis following uretero-sigmoidostomy, in other forms of acidosis due to organic acids or failure of renal hydrion and ammonium excretion, the [Cl] may be normal. Except in special cases, the [Cl] is perhaps the least valuable of the four basic electrolyte estimations on plasma; and inferences on acid-base disturbances are more reliably made from the plasma [HCO$_3$], [H], and P_{CO_2}.

The plasma *bicarbonate* lies between 25 and 29 mEq/l. in most normal people, though the 98 per cent range is from 24 to 31 mEq/l. (Wootton and King, 1953). The plasma [HCO$_3$] is low in metabolic acidosis and in respiratory alkalosis, and high in metabolic alkalosis and respiratory acidosis. The possible confusion between respiratory and metabolic or renal disturbances of acid-base balance can usually be resolved clinically, but I have known patients in whom dyspnoea closely simulated hyperpnoea or in whom hyperpnoea simulated voluntary hyperventilation; so that a final diagnosis of the character of the acid-base disturbance rested on the [H] of plasma. I have also seen patients in whom a raised plasma bicarbonate coincided with a normal plasma [K], but was nevertheless a pointer to K depletion, in that it fell to normal levels when alkaline salts of potassium were given.

Besides estimations of electrolyte concentrations themselves, concentrations of other plasma constituents may be helpful in assessing disturbances of body-fluid. Increase in the blood *urea* may draw attention to primary renal disease, or it may betoken so-called 'extrarenal uraemia' in which the renal circulation is depressed by general disease. In this way, attention may be called to primary sodium depletion, which may be associated with a blood urea of over 100 mg/100 ml; or to water depletion, in which the uraemia is more modest. Rapid changes in the *haemoglobin, haematocrit,* or *plasma proteins* are often related to sodium depletion or excess, but base-line values are often unknown, which limits the value of these estimations in the initial assessment of body-fluid disorders; serial measurements can help in the control of treatment. Apart from these acute secondary changes in plasma protein, the hypoproteinaemia of renal or hepatic disease is of course relevant to the development of sodium excess. Estimations of *plasma volume* are low in sodium depletion, but are scarcely necessary for diagnosis. Other biochemical estimations, such as calcium, phosphorus, bilirubin and so on, may be crucial in the investigation of the cause of a body-fluid disorder, but are not called for in the general assessment of body-fluid.

Urine. Apart from the general indications of disease afforded by routine qualitative testing, examination of the urine may be of special value in clarifying disturbances of body-fluid. The expected renal responses to change in body-fluid have been described in previous chapters; gross deviation from these may point to a renal cause of the disturbance, or to an abnormal balance of hormones acting on the kidneys. In this context, we would stress the importance of determining renal behaviour with respect to water and electrolytes, as opposed to the so-called 'discrete tests of renal function', such as inulin and PAH clearance. In saying this, no criticism is made of the value of these tests in special studies of renal physiology and pathology; but in the practical assessment of body-fluid, sufficient information on renal excretory function can be gained from the clearance of urea or creatinine, or even from a raised blood-urea concentration. On the other hand, abnormal renal tubular behaviour as a cause of body-fluid disturbance can occur with a normal blood urea, and will only be detected by observations on the urinary acidity and excretion of water and electrolytes. In any chronic disorder of body-fluid for which no extrarenal cause is apparent, a fresh specimen of urine should have the pH determined, and a 24-hour specimen of urine should be examined for its content of Na, K and Cl. Examination of the urine is less valuable in the assessment of acute electrolyte depletion. The semi-quantitative test for urinary chloride (Fantus, 1936) is sometimes recommended as a guide to the need for saline; but it is often misleading, either because of acid-base disturbances which dissociate the excretion of chloride from that of sodium, or more commonly, because of the post-operative retention of sodium and chloride in the absence of any depletion. The introduction of rapid methods of plasma analysis has, in my view, made this test obsolete; and its use in the post-operative period must tend to promote unnecessary treatment with saline fluid.

OTHER ESTIMATIONS

Occasional help in planning treatment can be obtained by estimating the electrolyte output over a 24-hour period in aspirated material, vomit, or fluid faeces; this unpleasant task is of course an integral part of balance experiments which give retrospective information on electrolyte deficits. Determination of total body-water, (Na) or (K) with isotopes is a method of assessing depletion which is independent of balance observations, but which is best used in conjunction with them. Neither of these assessments is of immediate practical value. At any rate, in the assessment of acute disorders of body-fluid they are both much inferior to the mundane procedure of weighing the patient once a day, or oftener. For example, simple weighing allowed Tinckler (1966) to establish that in the tropics 'insensible' losses of water ranged between 2 and 4 litres a day. An indication of adrenal mineralocorticoid activity is given by the electrolyte composition of sweat (Conn, 1949); this indication should be supplemented by hormone assay and observations on urinary electrolyte output. The Na/K ratio in faecal water, samplable in plastic sacs, is another index of mineralocorticoid activity (Wrong *et al*, 1961).

We have now considered, at least in outline, the categories of information on which diagnostic and therapeutic decisions must be based (such decisions in matters of fluid-balance are notably inter-dependent, and often final diagnosis depends on the response to treatment—'facio ut intelligam' is an apophthegm for the fluid-therapist). The 'trial and error' quality of fluid therapy, emphasized by Elkinton and Danowski (1955) would be endorsed by any who have had experience in it. This implies that the situation must be reassessed from day to day, and in acute problems at even more frequent intervals. The process of reassessment is made much more convenient by a well-organized, but simple, method of charting the relevant data. Such a scheme has been proposed by Preedy and Richardson (1956).

Principles of Treatment

The ultimate object of treatment is clearly to restore normal amount and composition of body-fluid. This may be accomplished eventually by cure of a remediable disease or by continued palliation of a persistent disease; but the ultimate curative treatment may only become possible after the immediate effects of gross fluid imbalance have been corrected by treatment specifically directed at water and electrolyte balance. In carrying out such treatment, attention has to be paid to:

(1) Maintenance of current fluid balance.

(2) Replacement of those day-to-day abnormal losses of water and electrolyte which cannot be quickly arrested.

(3) Correction of existing deficits and excesses.

(1) *The maintenance of current fluid balance* for short periods concerns mainly water (see p. 33). For most patients, 2 litres a day is adequate; larger amounts are needed in patients with fever or polyuria, and smaller amounts in patients with anuria or gross oliguria. The best method of administration, when possible, is by drinking; failing this, by indwelling small-bore gastric tube; and in patients who

cannot tolerate a tube, by intravenous 5 per cent glucose. For periods of artificial feeding longer than a few days, an adequate daily intake of water, electrolytes and food can be provided by 3 litres of milk given by stomach-tube, or by 2 litres with added casein hydrolysate and cream. Various proprietary foods have been specially designed for tube-feeding, but some of them are of high-protein content; this involves the excretion of considerable amounts of urea, and this in turn may demand more water than is supplied if the maker's recommendations for diluting the feeds are followed (Jones and Sachiari, 1963). The difficulties inherent in prolonged intravenous feeding have not yet been entirely solved, but considerable progress is being made. Jones and Peaston (1966) suggest that patients with acute illness of many kinds are commonly under-nourished, because of apathy and anorexia. They require a caloric intake of at least 2000/day, given orally or by gastric tube, and if necessary intravenously. If tube-feeding leads to diarrhoea, this may be controlled—paradoxically—by providing some 'roughage', such as methylcellulose. In the absence of adequate calories, protein hydrolysates have proved disappointing, because of the deviation of amino acids from protein synthesis to breakdown for energy-production, and also because of the considerable excretion of intravenously given amino acids in the urine. Blood and plasma are more satisfactory sources of intravenous protein. Alcohol, sucrose and fructose have been used as alternatives to glucose for intravenous feeding. Extracellular electrolyte can be given intravenously for maintenance by including in the solution sodium chloride in a concentration of 0.17 per cent or 29 mM/l., i.e. 'fifth-normal saline'. When there are no abnormal losses, potassium balance can be maintained on 50 mEq/day, and this should preferably be given by mouth, but can be given intravenously in a concentration of 25 mEq/l. in a 2-litre fluid intake; there may be some advantage in giving the K with phosphate, the main intracellular anion.

These general recommendations do not take account of body-size, and this is specially important in the case of children, reviewed by Darrow (1959). He bases his estimate of requirements primarily on the caloric intake, rather than on surface area. For each 100 calories consumed, he suggests an intake of 100 ml water, and 2–3 mEq of Na, K and Cl. The calorie intake is of the order of 1000 calories/sq. m of surface area; but is proportionally larger in the smaller, more rapidly growing, children.

(2) *Replacement of abnormal losses.* Obvious losses of electrolyte-containing fluid from the alimentary tract tend to produce acute depletion of body-fluid; the fluid lost should always be measured, and if possible analysed for [Na], [K] and [Cl] in a 24-hour specimen. If this information is available, the Na:K ratio and the Cl:HCO_3 ratio of the replacement fluid can be prescribed and given during the ensuing day. This presupposes a prompt biochemical service, and for most purposes it is sufficient to replace gastric losses with fluid which will provide some hydrion to replace that lost in the gastric juice; conversely, losses of alkaline intestinal fluid should be appropriately replaced. Suitable intravenous fluids for the volume-for-volume replacement of aspirated alimentary fluids have been suggested by Cooke and Crowley (1952).*

Occult losses of Na and K in the stools and urine may lead insidiously to chronic electrolyte depletion; once it has been recognized, this can be treated by oral electrolyte supplements. Measurement of the relevant output of electrolyte at different levels of intake is of great assistance in deciding the amount and composition of the supplements required for subsequent management; but it does not do away with the need for regular checks on plasma electrolyte concentrations in patients with chronic urinary or faecal electrolyte loss who are being maintained on supplements.

(3) *Correction of excesses and deficits.* General methods of treatment applicable to the correction of excesses and deficits of water, and of sodium, potassium and anions, have been outlined in previous chapters. In this section, the information previously given will not be repeated in detail, but we will attempt to outline the synthesis required for the treatment of combined disturbances of body-fluid.

---

* These fluids are:
'Gastric replacement fluid.' NH_4Cl 3.75 g/l., NaCl 3.7 g/l., KCl 1.3 g/l., i.e. [Na] 63, [K] 17, [NH_4] 70 and [Cl] 150 mEq/l.
'Intestinal replacement fluid.' Na lactate 5.6 g/l., NaCl 5.1 g/l., KCl 0.9 g/l., i.e. [Na] 138, [K] 12, [Cl] 100 and [lactate] 50 mEq/l.
In the gastric fluid, NH_4 is metabolized to urea$+H^+$, given adequate hepatic function; in the intestinal fluid, lactate is effectively a source of bicarbonate.

Little need be added to what has already been said of the treatment of *excesses* of water and electrolytes. In clinical terms, this means most commonly the treatment of generalized oedema, which has been described under the heading of 'sodium excess' (p. 67); this is of course a combined excess, since water, chloride and bicarbonate are all retained with sodium, but there is no need for separate attention to these subsidiary excesses. Isolated excesses of water (p. 37), of potassium (p. 103) and of hydrion (p. 121) have already been discussed.

The treatment of *depletion* of body-fluid, or of its separate constituents, is more complex, because of the interrelations between the different electrolytes, and the difficulties imposed by the effect of severe Na depletion on the circulation and renal function, and of severe K depletion on cellular function generally. There are indeed many patients with mild depletion of recent onset in whom treatment with a few litres of isotonic saline or of 5 per cent glucose is all that is required, depending on whether sodium depletion or water depletion is the more prominent; the finer adjustment of potassium balance and acid-base balance will be achieved by the kidneys when they are given enough fluid to work on. The really difficult problems are presented by those patients with very severe sodium depletion complicated by potassium depletion, and by acid-base imbalance; I have discussed the therapeutic difficulties in those particular patients elsewhere (Black, 1953). I would again emphasize the large amounts of sodium required, over 1000 mEq; the convenience of giving such large amounts as hypertonic solutions (5 per cent NaCl or molar Na lactate); and the necessity, when large amounts are given, of giving part of the infusion as lactate or bicarbonate rather than as chloride. Further experience (Black and Williams, 1962) has shown that hypertonic solutions of sodium, including lactate, have a place in the treatment of renal failure, when the amounts of Na required are smaller, but the dangers of over-loading with fluid are often more considerable, because of hypertension. Darrow (1959) has given hypertonic saline in paediatric practice, when severe Na depletion needed prompt treatment; this does not conflict with the value of '⅓ normal saline' for general maintenance of fluid intake in children. Merrill (1956) has pointed out that if patients are under treatment with digitalis, they may become more sensitive when given hypertonic infusions, because of hypokalaemia; this risk can be avoided by including potassium in the infusion. The state of peripheral circulatory failure may demand blood or plasma infusion, and sometimes the addition of vasoconstrictors (or vasodilators) to the intravenous drip. As renal function and urinary output improve, and as the plasma and E.C.F. expand in volume, hypokalaemia often develops, and demands the inclusion of potassium in the intravenous infusions, in concentrations up to 40 mEq/l. Fortunately, it is seldom necessary to make up the whole K deficit by the intravenous route, for the acute and dangerous symptoms of hypokalaemia disappear long before this has been done, and the bulk of the K deficit can then be made up by oral potassium.

A great many intravenous solutions for fluid therapy have been described, of which a rather complete account is given by Weisberg (1962). This situation leads to confusion, and it is better to gain experience in the use of only a few solutions. For patients who can retain oral medicaments, 0.5 per cent NaCl solution, capsules or tablets of NaCl or $NaHCO_3$, and a potassium mixture such as Mist. Pot. Cit. (N.F.) or tablets of KCl or $KHCO_3$ are available. For intravenous use, isotonic saline and glucose; 5 per cent saline with varying amounts of molar sodium lactate added; the 'gastric' and 'intestinal' solutions (p. 147); and a solution with 40 mEq of K and lactate, and 100 mEq of Na and Cl per litre are adequate for most purposes. There is no 'dose' of such preparations. The amount to be given has to be assessed from the initial clinical and biochemical observations, and reassessed from time to time by further observations, of which those concerning general well-being, the state of the circulation and the amount of urine formed are perhaps the most important. Neyzi et al (1958) have shown that fluid and electrolytes are better retained if the required amount is distributed throughout the day, rather than given in short infusions.

I have tried to make this final section on treatment an individual one, with little reference to other accounts of the matter. Of these, that of Elkinton and Danowski (1955) is particularly comprehensive and detailed; while Josephson (1961) and Weisberg (1962) give recent general reviews. A multiple-author survey, which does more justice to the detailed literature than is possible in the compilation of a single author, is now appearing (Comar and Bronner, 1960). The more clinical aspects are now being similarly dealt with in Bland (1963). Surgical problems have been specially discussed by Wilkinson (1960). The special problems of fluid therapy in paediatrics have been the subject of a symposium edited by Barness (1959).

This book is itself no more than a summary of what has become a very extensive body of information. Its purpose will have been served if it interests even a few of those who may read it, and especially if it should stimulate them either to study the benefits of practical attention to fluid balance, or to fill in one or two of the many gaps in theoretical knowledge. For the first of these objectives the key-reference is the book of Nature; for the second, a monograph of this size can only give a general outline of present information, and for a detailed survey of individual topics, those interested should consult recent review articles, of which a number are given in the list of references.

REFERENCES

(Reviews marked*)

ABER G.M., SAMPSON P.A., WHITEHEAD T.P. and BROOKE B.N. (1962) The role of chloride in the correction of alkalosis associated with potassium depletion. *Lancet* 2, 1028

ACHOR R.W.P. and SMITH L.A. (1955) Nutritional deficiency syndrome with diarrhoea resulting in hypopotassemia, muscle degeneration, and renal insufficiency; report of case with recovery. *Proc. Mayo Clin.* 30, 207

ADAMS R.D., DENNY-BROWN D. and PEARSON C.M. (1953) *Diseases of Muscle.* London, 1953

ADLER S., ROY A. and RELMAN A.S. (1965) Intracellular acid-base regulation. II. The interaction between CO_2 tension and extracellular bicarbonate in the determination of muscle cell pH. *J. clin. Invest.* 44, 21

AIRD I., MILNE M.D. and MUEHRCKE R.C. (1956) Potassium-losing nephritis. *Brit. med. J.* 1, 1042

ALBRINK M.J., HALD P.M., MAN E.B. and PETERS J.P. (1955) The displacement of serum water by the lipids of hyperlipemic serum. A new method for the rapid determination of serum water. *J. clin. Invest.* 34, 1483

ANDERSSON B. and McCANN S.M. (1955) A further study of polydipsia evoked by hypothalamic stimulation in the goat. *Acta physiol. Scand.* 33, 333

ANDRES R., CADER G., GOLDMAN P. and ZIERLER K.L. (1957) Net potassium movement between resting muscle and plasma in man in the basal state and during the night. *J. clin. Invest.* 36, 723

ANDRIOLE V.T. and EPSTEIN F.H. (1965) Prevention of pyelonephritis by water diuresis; evidence for the role of medullary hypertonicity in promoting renal infection. *J. clin. Invest.* 44, 73

ARDAILLOU R. and RICHET G. (1966) Production d'ions H^+ à partir des phospholipides des oeufs. *Rev. Franç d'étud. clin. biol.* 11, 519

ARIEL I.M. (1954) Chloridorrhoea: syndrome associated with diarrhoea and potassium deficiency. *Arch. Surg.* 68, 105

ASANO S., KATO E., YAMAUCHI M., OZAWA Y., IWASA M., WADA T. and HASEGAWA, H. (1965) The mechanism of the acidosis caused by infusion of saline solution. *Lancet.* 1, 1245

ASTRUP P., JORGENSEN K., ANDERSEN O.S. and ENGEL K. (1960) The acid-base metabolism. A new approach. *Lancet* 1, 1035

ATKINS E.L. and SCHWARTZ W.B. (1962) Factors governing correction of the alkalosis associated with potassium deficiency; the critical role of chloride in the recovery process. *J. clin. Invest.* **41,** 218

BABA W.I., TUDHOPE G.R. and WILSON G.M. (1962) Triamterene, a new diuretic drug. *Brit. med. J.* **2,** 756 and 760

BAGSHAWE K.D. (1960) Hypokalaemia, carcinoma, and Cushing's syndrome. *Lancet* **2,** 284

BAKER D.R., SCHRADER W.H. and HITCHCOCK C.R. (1964) Small-bowel ulceration apparently associated with thiazide and potassium therapy. *J. Amer. med. Ass.* **190,** 586

BANYAJATI C., KEOPLUG M., BIESEL W.R., GANGAROSA E.J., SPRINZ H. and SIT-PRIJA V. (1960) Acute renal failure in Asiatic cholera. Clinicopathologic correlations with acute tubular necrosis and hypokalaemic nephropathy. *Ann. intern. Med.* **52,** 960

BARLOW E.D. and DE WARDENER H.E. (1959) Compulsive water drinking. *Quart. J. Med.* **28,** 235

BARNES B.A., GORDON E.B. and COPE O. (1957) Skeletal muscle analyses in health and in certain metabolic disorders. I. The method of analysis and the values in normal muscle. *J. clin. Invest.* **36,** 1239

★ BARNESS L.A. (editor) Symposium on fluid and electrolyte problems. *Pediat. Clin. N. Amer.* **6,** 1–336

BARRACLOUGH M.A. (1966) Sodium and water depletion with acute malignant hypertension. *Amer. J. Med.* **40,** 265

BARRACLOUGH M.A., JONES J.J. and LEE J. (1966) Production of vasopressin by anaplastic oat cell carcinoma of the bronchus. *Clin. Sci.* **31,** 135

BARTER J. and FORBES G.B. (1963) Correlation of potassium-40 data with anthropometric measurements. *Ann. N.Y. Acad. Sci.* **110,** 264

BARTTER F.C. (1958) The physiological control of aldosterone secretion. *Proc. Roy. Soc. Med.* **51,** 201

BARTTER F.C. and FOURMAN P. (1957) A non-renal effect of adrenal cortical steroids on potassium metabolism. *J. clin. Invest.* **36,** 872

BARTTER F.C., MILLS I.H. and GANN D.S. (1960) Increase in aldosterone secretion by carotid artery constriction in the dog, and its prevention by thyrocarotid arterial junction denervation. *J. clin. Invest.* **39,** 1330

BARTTER F.C., PRONOVE P., GILL J.R. and MacCARDLE R.C. (1962) Hyperplasia of the juxtaglomerular complex with hyperaldosteronism and hypokalemic alkalosis. A new syndrome. *Amer. J. Med.* **33,** 811

BARTTER, F.C. and SCHWARTZ, W.B. (1967) The syndrome of inappropriate secretion of antidiuretic hormone. *Amer. J. Med.* **42,** 790

BAUM G.L., DICK M.M. BLUM A., KAUPE A. and CARBALLO J. (1959) Factors involved in digitalis sensitivity in chronic pulmonary insufficiency. *Amer. Heart J.* **57,** 460

BAYLISS, R.I.S. (1966) Corticosteroids in heart disease. *Brit. med. J.* **2,** 721

★ BELLET S. (1955) The ECG in electrolyte imbalance. *Arch. intern. Med.* **96,** 618

* BERGER E.Y. (1960) Intestinal absorption and excretion. Chapter 8 in *Mineral Metabolism*, ed. C.L. Comar and F. Bronner. New York, 1960

BERGSTROM W.H. (1956) The skeleton as an electrolyte reservoir. *Metabolism* **5**, 433

BERLINER R.W., KENNEDY T.J. and ORLOFF J. (1951) Relationship between acidification of the urine and potassium metabolism. *Amer. J. Med.* **11**, 274

BERLYNE G.M. (1961) Distal tubular function in chronic hydronephrosis. *Quart. J. Med.* **30**, 339

BETHUNE J.E. and NELSON D.H. (1965) Hyponatremia in hypopituitarism. *New Eng. J. Med.* **272**, 771

BLACK D.A.K. (1952) *Sodium Metabolism in Health and Disease*. Oxford, 1952

BLACK D.A.K. (1953) Body fluid depletion. *Lancet* **1**, 305 and 353

* BLACK D.A.K. (1962) *Renal Disease*. Oxford, 1962

BLACK D.A.K. (1965) Renal rete mirabile. *Lancet* **2**, 1141.

*BLACK D.A.K. (1967) *Renal Disease* (2nd edn.). Oxford, 1967

BLACK D.A.K., DAVIES H.E.F. and EMERY E.W (1955) The disposal of radioactive potassium injected intravenously. *Lancet* **1**, 1097

BLACK D.A.K. and EMERY E.W. (1957) Tubular secretion of potassium. *Brit. med. Bull.* **13**, 7

BLACK D.A.K., McCANCE R.A. and YOUNG W.F. (1944) A study of dehydration by means of balance experiments. *J. Physiol.* **102**, 406

BLACK D.A.K. and MILNE M.D. (1952) Experimental potassium depletion in man. *Clin. Sci.* **11**, 397

BLACK D.A.K. and WILLIAMS R.T. (1962) The use of hypertonic saline in patients with renal failure. *Quart. J. Med.* **31**, 57

BLAHD W.H. and BASSETT S.H. (1953) Potassium deficiency in man. *Metabolism* **2**, 218

BLAIR-WEST J.R., COGHLAN J.P., DENTON D.A., GODING J.R., ORCHARD E., SCOGGINS B., WINTOUR M. and WRIGHT R.D. (1966) Mechanisms regulating aldosterone secretion during Na deficiency. *Symposium on angiotensin and aldosterone*, III. International Congress of Nephrology, Washington, 1966

BLAKE W.D. (1955) Pathways of adrenaline action on renal function with observations on a blood pressure reflex regulating water and electrolyte excretion. *Amer. J. Physiol.* **181**, 399

* BLAND J.H. (1963) *Clinical Metabolism of Water and Electrolytes*. Philadelphia, 1963

BLEICH H.L. and SCHWARTZ W.B. (1966) Tris buffer (THAM). *New Eng. J. Med.* **274**, 782

BOLING E.A. and LIPKIND J.B. (1963) Body composition and serum electrolyte concentrations. *J. appl. Physiol.* **18**, 943

BORST J.G.G. (1948) The maintenance of an adequate cardiac output by the regulation of the urinary excretion of water and sodium chloride; an essential factor in the genesis of oedema. *Acta med. Scand. Supp.* **207**

BRACKETT N.C., COHEN J.J. and SCHWARTZ W.B. (1965) Carbon dioxide titration curve of normal man. *New Eng. J. Med.* **272**, 6

BRAIN W.R. (1962) *Diseases of the Nervous System*, 6th edn. Oxford, 1962

BRENNER O. (1959) Electrolyte disturbances in heart failure. P. 182 in *Clinical Effects of Electrolyte Disturbances*, ed. E.J. Ross. London, 1959

BRICKER N.S., SCHWAYRI E.I., REARDAN J.B., KELLOG G., MERRILL, J.P. and HOLMES J.H. (1957) An abnormality in renal function resulting from urinary tract obstruction. *Amer. J. Med.* 23, 554

BRICKER N.S. (1967) Obstructive nephropathy. Chapter in *Renal Disease* (2nd edn.), ed. D.A.K. Black. Oxford, 1967

BROD J. and FEJFAR Z. (1950) The origin of oedema in heart failure. *Quart. J. Med.* 19, 187

BROWN J.J., DAVIES D.L., LEVER A.F., McPHERSON D. and ROBERTSON J.I.S. (1966) Plasma renin concentration in relation to changes in posture. *Clin. Sci.* 30, 279

BROWN J.J., DAVIES D.L., LEVER A.F. and ROBERTSON J.I.S. (1963) Influence of sodium loading and sodium depletion on plasma-renin in man. *Lancet* 2, 278

BROWN J.J. and PEART W.S. (1962) The effect of angiotensin on urine flow and electrolyte excretion in hypertensive patients. *Clin. Sci.* 22, 1

BRUNNER F.P., RECTOR F.C. and SELDIN D.W. (1966) Mechanics of glomerulo-tubular balance. II. *J. clin. Invest.* 45, 603

BULL G.M., CARTER A.B. and LOWE K.G. (1953) Hyperpotassaemic paralysis. *Lancet* 2, 60

BULL G.M., JOEKES A.M. and LOWE K.G. (1950) Renal function studies in acute tubular necrosis. *Clin. Sci.* 9, 379

BUNGE G. (1873) Über die bedeutung des kochsalzes und das verhalten der kalisalz im menschlichen organismus. *Z. Biol.* 9, 104

BURNETT C.H., BURROWS B.A., COMMONS R.R. and TOWERY B.T. (1950) Studies of alkalosis: II Electrolyte abnormalities in alkalosis resulting from pyloric obstruction. *J. clin. Invest.* 29, 175

BURNETT C.H., COMMONS R.R., ALBRIGHT F. and HOWARD J.E. (1948) Syndrome characterized by hypercalcemia, calcinosis, and renal insufficiency following prolonged intake of calcium and alkali. *J. clin. Endocrinol.* 8, 584

CAMERON J.M. and DAYAN A.D. (1966) Association of brain damage with therapeutic abortion induced by amniotic fluid replacement: report of two cases. *Brit. med. J.* 1, 1010

CAMPBELL W.A.B. (1955) Potassium levels in exchange transfusion. *Arch. Dis. Childh.* 30, 513

CAMPBELL E.J.M. (1962) RIpH. *Lancet* 1, 681

* CAMPBELL E.J.M. (1963) Chapter on 'Respiration' in *Clinical Physiology*, ed. E.J.M. Campbell, J. Dickinson and J.D.H. Slater. Blackwell, Oxford, 1963

CAMPBELL E.J.M. and HOWELL J.B.L. (1960) Simple rapid methods of estimating arterial and mixed venous P_{CO_2}. *Brit. med. J.* 1, 458

CANNON P.J., HEINEMANN H.O., ALBERT M.S., LARAGH J.H. and WINTERS R.W. (1965) 'Contraction' alkalosis after diuresis of edematous patients with ethacrynic acid. *Ann. intern. Med.* 62, 979

CANNON P.R., FRAZIER L.E. and HUGHES R.H. (1952) Influence of potassium on tissue protein synthesis. *Metabolism* **1,** 49

CANNON P.R., FRAZIER L.E. and HUGHES R.H. (1953) Sodium as a toxic ion in potassium deficiency. *Metabolism* **2,** 297

CARONE F.A. and COOKE R.E. (1953) Effect of potassium deficiency on gastric secretion in the rat. *Amer. J. Physiol.* **172,** 684

CARPENTER C.C.J., MITRA P.P., SACK R.B., DANS P.E., WELLS S.A. and CHAUD-HURI R.N. (1965) Clinical evaluation of fluid requirements in Asiatic cholera. *Lancet* **1,** 726

CARTER N.W., RECTOR F.C. and SELDIN D.W. (1961) Hyponatremia in cerebral disease resulting from the inappropriate secretion of antidiuretic hormone. *New Eng. J. Med.* **264,** 67

CARTER N.W., RECTOR F.C. and SELDIN D.W. (1967) Measurement of intracellular pH of skeletal muscle with pH-sensitive glass micro-electrodes. *J. clin. Invest.* **46,** 920

CARTER N.W., SELDIN D.W. and TENG H.C. (1959) Tissue and renal response to chronic respiratory acidosis. *J. clin. Invest.* **38,** 949

CAYLEY F.E. DE W. (1950) Potassium deficiency in p-aminosalicyclic acid therapy. *Lancet* **1,** 447

CHAMBERLAIN M.J. (1964) Emergency treatment of hyperkalaemia. *Lancet* **1,** 464

CHANDLER G.N., HETHERINGTON C., STEPHENSON A.N. and ATKINSON M. (1961) Potassium replacement therapy. *Gut* **2,** 186

CHRISTY N.P. and LARAGH J.H. (1961) Pathogenesis of hypokalemic alkalosis in Cushing's syndrome. *New Eng. J. Med.* **265,** 1083

CLARKSON B., THOMPSON D., HORWITH M., LUCKEY E.H. (1960) Cyclical edema and shock due to increased capillary permeability. *Amer. J. Med.* **29,** 193

CLEMENTSEN H.J. (1962) Potassium therapy. A break with tradition. *Lancet* **2,** 175

CHINARD F.P. and ENNS T. (1955) Relative renal excretion patterns of sodium ion, chloride ion, urea, water, and glomerular substances. *Amer. J. Physiol.* **182,** 247

CLARKE E., EVANS B.M., MACINTYRE I. and MILNE M.D. (1955) Acidosis in experimental electrolyte depletion. *Clin. Sci.* **14,** 421

CLAYTON-JONES E. (1953) Water intoxication. *Lancet* **1,** 549

COCHRAN R.T. (1963) Pulmonary insufficiency and hypercapnia complicated by potassium-responsive alkalosis. *New Eng. J. Med.* **268,** 521

COGGINS C.H. and LEAF A. (1967) Diabetes insipidus. *Amer. J. Med.* **42,** 807

COHEN J., SCHWARTZ R. and WALLACE W.M. (1952) Lesions of epiphyseal cartilage and skeletal muscle in rats on a diet deficient in potassium. *Arch. Path.* **54,** 119

COHEN J.J. and SCHWARTZ W.B. (1966) Evaluation of acid-base equilibrium in pulmonary insufficiency. *Amer. J. Med.* **41,** 163

COLLIER C.R. (1956) Determination of mixed venous CO_2 tension by rebreathing. *J. appl. Physiol.* **9,** 25

CONN J.W. (1949) Electrolyte composition of sweat; clinical implications as index of adrenal cortical function. *Arch. intern. Med.* **83,** 416

CONN J.W. (1961) Aldosteronism and hypertension: primary aldosteronism versus hypertensive disease with secondary aldosteronism. *Arch. intern. Med.* **107,** 813

CONN J.W., FAJANS S.S., LOUIS L.H., STREETEN D.H.P. and JOHNSON R.D. (1957) Intermittent aldosteronism in periodic paralysis. *Lancet* **1,** 802

CONN J.W. (1955) Primary aldosteronism. *J. Lab. Clin. Med.* **45,** 661

CONN J.W. and JOHNSON R.D. (1956) Kaliopenic nephropathy. *Amer. J. clin. Nutrit.* **4,** 523

COOKE A.M. (1932) Alkalosis occurring in alkaline treatment of peptic ulcers. *Quart. J. Med.* **1,** 527

COOKE R.E. and CROWLEY L.G. (1952) Replacement of gastric and intestinal fluid losses in surgery. *New Eng. J. Med.* **246,** 637

COOKE R.E., SEGAR W.E., CHEEK D.B., COVILLE F.E. and DARROW D.C. (1952) The extrarenal correction of alkalosis associated with potassium deficiency. *J. clin. Invest.* **31,** 798

COOKE R.E., SEGAR W.E., REED C., ETZWILER D.D., VITA M., BRUSILOW S. and DARROW D.C. (1954) The role of potassium in the prevention of alkalosis. *Amer. J. Med.* **17,** 180

COPE C.L. (1936) Alkali poisoning. A danger in the treatment of peptic ulcer. *Brit. med. J.* **2,** 914

COPE C.L., HARWOOD M. and PEARSON J. (1962) Aldosterone secretion in hypertensive disease. *Brit. med. J.* **1,** 659

COPPAGE W.S., ISLAND D.P., COONER A.E. and LIDDLE G.W. (1962) The metabolism of aldosterone in normal subjects and in patients with hepatic cirrhosis. *J. clin. Invest.* **41,** 1672

COPPEN A., SHAW D.M. and MANGONI A. (1962) Total exchangeable sodium in depressive illness. *Brit. med. J.* **2,** 295

CORT J.H. (1963a) On the use of studies *in vitro* in the transport of electrolytes and water. Chapter 5 in *Clinical Metabolism of Water and Electrolytes*, ed. J.H. Bland. Philadelphia, 1963

CORT J.H. (1963b) Relation of the central nervous system to water and electrolyte metabolism: physiologic and clinical aspects. Chapter 19 in Bland.

COULSON R.A. HERNANDEZ T. and DESSAUER H.G. (1950) Alkaline tide of the alligator. *Proc. Soc. Exp. Biol. N.Y.* **74,** 866

CRAWFORD J.D., KENNEDY G.C. and HILL L.E. (1960) Clinical results of treatment of diabetes insipidus with drugs of the chlorothiazide series. *New Eng. J. Med.* **262,** 737

CROCKETT D.J. (1956) The protein levels of oedema fluids. *Lancet* **2,** 1179

DAHL L.K. (1958) Salt intake and salt need. *New Eng. J. Med.* **258,** 1152

DANOWSKI T.S., ELKINTON J.R., BURROWS, B.A. and WINKLER A.W. (1948) Exchanges of sodium and potassium in familial periodic paralysis. *J. clin. Invest.* **27,** 65

DANOWSKI T.S., FERGUS E.B. and MATEER F.M. (1955) The low salt syndromes. *Ann. intern. Med.* **43,** 643

DANOWSKI T.S. and NABARRO J.D.N. (1965) Hyperosmolar and other types of non-ketoacidotic coma in diabetes. *Diabetes.* **14,** 162.

DARROW D.C. (1945) Body-fluid physiology: relation of tissue composition to problems of water and electrolyte balance. *New Eng. J. Med.* **233,** 91

DARROW D.C. (1946) The retention of electrolyte during recovery from severe dehydration due to diarrhoea. *J. Pediat.* **28,** 515

DARROW D.C. (1950) Body-fluid physiology: the role of potassium in clinical disturbances of body water and electrolytes. *New Eng. J. Med.* **242,** 978

* DARROW D.C. (1959) The physiologic basis for estimating requirements for parenteral fluids. *Pediat. Clin. N. Amer.* **6,** 29

DARROW D.C. and YANNET H. (1935) Changes in distribution of body water accompanying increase and decrease in extracellular electrolyte. *J. clin. Invest,* **14,** 266

DAUGHADAY W.H., LIPICKY R.J. and RASINSKI D.C. (1962) Lactic acidosis as a cause of nonketotic acidosis in diabetic patients. *New. Eng. J. Med.* **267,** 1010

DAVIDSON D.G., LEVINSKY N.G. and BERLINER R.W. (1957). Maintenance of potassium excretion despite reduction of glomerular filtration during sodium diuresis. *J. clin. Invest.* **36,** 882

DAVIDSON L.A.G., FLEAR C.T.G. and DONALD K.W. (1960) Transient amino-aciduria in severe potassium depletion. *Brit. med. J.* **1,** 911

DAVIES C.E. and KILPATRICK J.A. (1951) Renal circulation in 'low output' and 'high output' heart failure. *Clin. Sci.* **10,** 53

DAVIES H.E.F., JEPSON R.P. and BLACK D.A.K. (1956) Some metabolic sequels of gastric surgery in patients with and without pyloric stenosis. *Clin. Sci.* **15,** 61

DAVIS J.O., CARPENTER C.C.J., AYERS C.R., HOLMAN J.E. and BAHN R.C. (1961) Evidence for secretion of an aldosterone-stimulating hormone by the kidney. *J. clin. Invest.* **40,** 684

DAVIS J.O., JOHNSTON C.I., HOWARDS, S.S. and WRIGHT F.S. (1967) Humoral factors in the regulation of renal sodium excretion. *Fed. Proc.* **26,** 60

DAVIS J.O., OLICHNEY M.J., BROWN T.C. and BINNION P.F. (1965) Metabolism of aldosterone in several experimental situations with altered aldosterone secretion. *J. clin. Invest.* **44,** 1433

DAVIS J.O., URQUHART J. and HIGGINS J.T. (1963) The effects of alterations of plasma sodium and potassium concentrations on aldosterone secretion. *J. clin. Invest.* **42,** 597

DEAN R.B. (1951) Theories of electrolyte equilibrium in muscle. *Biol. Symposia.* **3,** 331

DEANE N., ZIFF M. and SMITH H.W. (1952) The distribution of total body chloride in man. *J. clin. Invest.* **31,** 220

DE DEUXCHAINES C.N., COLLET R.A., BUSSET R. and MACH R.S. (1961) Exchange-able potassium in wasting, amyotrophy, heart-disease, and cirrhosis of the liver. *Lancet* **1,** 681

DE GRAEFF J. and LIPS J.B. (1957) Hypernatremia in diabetes mellitus. *Acta med. scand.* **157,** 72

DE GRAEFF J., STRUYVENBERG A. and LAMEIJER L.D.F. (1964) The role of chloride in hypokalemic alkalosis. *Amer. J. Med.* **37,** 778

DENTON D.A., WYNN V., McDONALD I.R. and SIMON S. (1951) Renal regulation of the extracellular fluid. *Acta med. Scand.* Supp. **261**

DENTON D.A. (1965) Evolutionary aspects of the emergence of aldosterone secretion and salt appetite. *Physiol. Rev.* **45,** 245

★ DE WARDENER H.E. (1962) Polyuria. Chapter 25 in *Renal Disease*, ed. D.A.K. Black. Blackwell, Oxford, 1962

DE WARDENER H.E. and HERXHEIMER A.W. (1957) The effect of a high water intake on the kidney's ability to concentrate the urine in man. *J. Physiol.* **139,** 42

DI GIOVANNI C. and BIRKHEAD N.C. (1964) Effect of minimal dehydration on orthostatic tolerance following short-term bed-rest. *Aerospace Med.* **35,** 225

DILL D.B. (1938) *Life, Heat and Altitude.* Cambridge, Mass., 1938

DIXON M. and WEBB E.C. (1964) *Enzymes,* 2nd edn. London, 1964

DOAK P.B. and EYRE K.E.D. (1961) Carbohydrate and sodium metabolism in periodic paralysis. *Brit. med. J.* **2,** 549

DOCK W. (1946) Sodium depletion as a therapeutic procedure; the value of ion exchange resins in withdrawing sodium from the body. *Trans. Ass. Amer. Physcns.* **59,** 282

DOLLERY C.T., SHACKMAN R. and SHILLINGFORD J. (1959) Malignant hypertension and hypokalaemia: cured by nephrectomy. *Brit. med. J.* **2,** 1367

DONALD K.W. (1955) Drowning. *Brit. med. J.* **2,** 155

DONALDSON V.H. and EVANS R.R. (1963) A biochemical abnormality in hereditary angioneurotic edema. *Amer. J. Med.* **35,** 37

DORMANDY T.L. (1966) Body pH. *Lancet* **1,** 755

DRESCHER A.N., TALBOT N.B., MEARA P.A., TERRY M. and CRAWFORD J.D. (1958) A study of the effects of excessive potassium intake upon body potassium stores. *J. clin. Invest.* **37,** 1316

DUGUID H., SIMPSON R.G. and STOWERS J.M. (1961) Accidental hypothermia. *Lancet* **2,** 1213

DUNNING M.F. and PLUM F. (1956) Potassium depletion by enemas. *Amer. J. Med.* **20,** 789

ECKEL R.E., NORRIS J.E.C. and POPE C.E. (1958) Basic amino acids as intracellular cations in K deficiency. *Amer. J. Physiol.* **193,** 644

EDELMAN, I.S. BOGOROCH R. and PORTER G.A. (1964) On the mechanism of action of aldosterone on sodium transport: the role of protein synthesis. *Proc. Nat. Acad. Sci. U.S.A.* **50,** 1169

EDELMAN I.S., HALEY H.B., SCHLOERB P.R., SHELDON D.B., FRIIS-HANSEN B.J., STOLL G. and MOORE F.D. (1952) Further observations on total body-water. I. Normal values throughout the life span. *Surg., Gynecol., Obstet,* **95,** 1

EDELMAN I.S., JAMES A.H., BADEN H. and MOORE F.D. (1954) Electrolyte composition of bone and the penetration of radiosodium and deuterium oxide into dog and human bone. *J. clin. Invest.* **33**, 122

★ EDELMAN I.S. and LEIBMAN J. (1959) Anatomy of body-water and electrolytes. *Amer. J. Med.* **27**, 256

EDELMAN I.S., LEIBMAN J., O'MEARA M.P. and BIRKENFELD L.W. (1958) Interrelations between serum sodium concentration, serum osmolality, and total exchangeable sodium, total exchangeable potassium and total body water. *J. clin. Invest.* **37**, 1236

EDMONDS C.J. (1960) An aldosterone antagonist and diuretics in the treatment of chronic oedema and ascites. *Lancet* **1**, 509

ELIAKIM M., ROSENBERG S.M. and BRAUN K. (1959) Electrocardiographic changes following the administration of hypertonic saline to dogs. *Amer. Heart J.* **58**, 97

ELITHORN A., BRIDGES P.K., LOBBAN M.C. and TREDRE B.E. (1966) Observations on some diurnal rhythms in depressive illness. *Brit. med. J.* **2**, 1620

ELKINTON J.R. and DANOWSKI I.S. (1955) *The Body Fluids: Basic Physiology and Practical Therapeutics.* London, 1955

ELKINTON J.R., DANOWSKI T.S. and WINKLER A.W. (1946) Hemodynamic changes in salt depletion and in dehydration. *J. clin. Invest.* **25**, 120

ELKINTON J.R., HUTH E.J., WEBSTER G.D. and McCANCE R.A. (1960) The renal excretion of hydrogen ion in renal tubular acidosis. I. Quantitative assessment of the response to ammonium chloride as an acid load. *Amer. J. Med.* **29**, 554

★ ELKINTON J.R., McCURDY D.K. and BUCKALEW V.M. (1967) Chapter on Hydrogen ion and the kidney in *Renal Disease*, 2nd edn., ed. D.A.K. Black. Oxford, 1967

ENGEL F.L. and JAEGER C. (1954) Dehydration with hypernatremia, hyperchloremia and azotemia complicating nasogastric tube feeding. *Amer. J. Med.* **17**, 196

ENGEL F.L., MARTIN S.P. and TAYLOR H. (1949) On relation of potassium to neurological manifestations of hypocalcemic tetany. *Bull. J. Hopk. Hosp.* **84**, 285

EPSTEIN S.E. and BRAUNWALD E. (1966) The effect of beta adrenergic blockade on patterns of urinary sodium excretion. *Ann. intern. Med.* **65**, 20

ERULKAR S.D. and MAREN T.H. (1961) Carbonic anhydrase and the inner ear. *Nature, Lond.* **189**, 459

EVANS B.M., HUGHES-JONES N.C., MILNE M.D. and YELLOWLEES H. (1953) Ion-exchange resins in the treatment of anuria. *Lancet* **2**, 792

EVANS B.M., MACINTYRE I., MACPHERSON C.R., and MILNE M.D. (1957) Alkalosis in sodium and potassium depletion (with special reference to organic acid excretion). *Clin. Sci.* **16**, 53

FANTUS B. (1936) Fluid postoperatively. *J. Amer. med. Ass.* **107**, 14

★ FARRELL G. (1958) Regulation of aldosterone secretion. *Physiol. Rev.* **38**, 709

FAWCETT J.K. and WYNN V. (1956) Variations of plasma electrolyte and total-protein levels in the individual. *Brit med. J.* **2**, 582

FERREBEE J.W., PARKER D., CARNES W.H., GERITY M.K., ATCHLEY D.W. and LOEB R.F. (1941) Certain effects of desoxycorticosterone: development of 'diabetes insipidus' and replacement of muscle potassium by sodium in normal dogs. *Amer. J. Physiol.* **135,** 230

FERRIS T., KASHGARIAN M., LEVITIN H., BRANDT I. and EPSTEIN F.H. (1961) Renal tubular acidosis and renal potassium wasting acquired as a result of hypercalcemic nephropathy. *New Eng. J. Med.* **265,** 924

FINBERG L. (1957) Experimental studies of the mechanisms producing hypocalcemia in hypernatremic states. *J. clin. Invest.* **36,** 434

FINBERG L., KILEY J. and LUTTRELL C.N. (1963) Mass accidental salt poisoning in infancy. *J. Amer. med. Ass.* **184,** 187

FINCH C.A., SAWYER C.G. and FLYNN J.M. (1946) Clinical syndrome of potassium intoxication. *Amer. J. Med.* **1,** 337

FISCH C., MARTZ B.L. and PRIEBE F.H. (1960) Enhancement of potassium-induced atrioventricular block by toxic doses of digitalis drugs. *J. clin. Invest.* **39,** 1885

FISCHER D.A., HUFFMAN E.R. and BLOUNT S.G. (1959) Massive edema due to bilateral incomplete renal artery occlusion. *Amer. J. Med.* **26,** 646

FISHBERG A.M. (1954) *Hypertension and Nephritis,* 5th edn. London, 1955

FISHMAN A.P., MAXWELL M.H., CROWDER C.H. and MORALES P. (1951) Kidney function in cor pulmonale. *Circulation* **3,** 703

FLEAR C.T.G. and CLARKE R. (1955) The influence of blood loss and blood transfusion upon changes in the metabolism of water, electrolytes and nitrogen following civilian trauma. *Clin. Sci.* **14,** 575

FOLCH-PI J., LEES M. and SLOANE-STANLEY G.H. (1957) The role of acidic lipides in the electrolytic balance of the nervous system of mammals. In *Metabolism of the Nervous System,* ed. D. Richter. London, 1957

FOLLIS R.H., ORENT-KEILES E. and McCOLLUM E.V. (1941) The production of cardiac and renal lesions in rats by a diet extremely deficient in potassium. *Amer. J. Path.* **18,** 29

FORBES G.B. and LEWIS A.M. (1956) Total sodium, potassium and chloride in adult man. *J. clin. Invest.* **35,** 596

FORBES G.B. and McCOORD A. (1965) Bone sodium as a function of serum sodium in rats. *Amer. J. Physiol.* **209,** 830

FORBES G.B. and PERLEY A. (1951) Estimation of total body sodium by isotope dilution. *J. clin. Invest.* **30,** 558

FORRESTER T.M. and SHIRRIFFS G.G. (1965) Frusemide and bendrofluazide in healthy subjects. *Lancet* **1,** 409

FOURMAN P. (1952) Effects of methyl testosterone and deoxycortone on electrolytes. *Clin. Sci.* **11,** 387

FOURMAN P. (1954a) Depletion of potassium induced in man with an exchange resin. *Clin. Sci.* **13,** 93

FOURMAN P. (1954b) Experimental observations on the tetany of potassium deficiency. *Lancet* **2,** 525

FOURMAN P. (1962) The adrenal cortex and the kidney. Chapter 25 in *Renal Disease,* ed. D.A.K. Black. Blackwell, Oxford, 1962

FOURMAN P. and LEESON P. (1959) Thirst and polyuria. *Lancet* **1**, 268

FOX C.L. and SLOBODY L.B. (1951) Tissue changes in the nephrotic syndrome: demonstration of potassium depletion. *Pediatrics* **7**, 186

FROMAN C. and CRAMPTON SMITH A. (1966) Hyperventilation associated with low pH of cerebrospinal fluid after intracranial haemorrhage. *Lancet* **1**, 780

FROST P.M. and SMITH J.L. (1953) Influence of potassium salts on efficiency of parenteral protein alimentation in the surgical patient. *Metabolism* **2**, 529

FUISZ R.G. (1963) Hyponatremia. *Medicine, Baltimore* **42**, 149

FULOP M. and DRAPKIN A. (1965) Potassium-depletion syndrome secondary to nephropathy apparently caused by 'outdated tetracycline'. *New Eng. J. Med.* **272**, 986

FURMAN K.I. (1965) Effects of muscular exercise on the dynamic patterns of sweat electrolyte secretion during heat stress exposures. *S. Afr. J. med. Sci.* **30**, 115

FURMAN K.I. and BEER G. (1963) Dynamic changes in sweat electrolyte composition induced by heat stress as an indication of acclimatization and aldosterone activity. *Clin. Sci.* **24**, 7.

GABUZDA G.J. (1962) Hepatic coma: clinical considerations, pathogenesis, and management. *Adv. intern. Med.* **11**, 1

GAMBLE J.L. (1946-47) Physiological information gained from studies on the life raft ration. *Harvey Lect.* **42**, 247

GAMBLE J.L. (1951) *Companionship of Water and Electrolytes in the Organization of Body Fluids.* Stanford, 1951

GAMBLE J.L. (1954) *Chemical Anatomy, Physiology, and Pathology of Extracellular Fluid.* Cambridge, Mass. 1954 (6th edn.)

GARDNER L.I., TALBOT N.B., COOK C.D., BERMAN H. and URIBE C. (1950) The effect of potassium deficiency on carbohydrate metabolism. *J. Lab. Clin. Med.* **35**, 592

GAUDINO M. and LEVITT M.F. (1949) Influence of the adrenal cortex on body water distribution and renal function. *J. clin. Invest.* **28**, 1487

GAUER O.H. and HENRY J.P. (1963) Circulatory basis of fluid volume control. *Physiol. Rev.* **43**, 423

GIBSON L.E. and COOKE R.E. (1959) A test for concentration of electrolytes in sweat in cystic fibrosis of the pancreas, utilizing pilocarpine by iontophoresis. *Pediatrics*, **23**, 545

GIEBISCH G., BERGER L. and PITTS R.F. (1955) The extrarenal response to acute acid-base disturbance of respiratory origin. *J. clin. Invest.* **34**, 231

GILBERT G.J. and GLASER G.H. (1961) On the nervous system integration of water and salt metabolism. *Arch. Neurol.* **5**, 179

GIPSTEIN, R.M. and BOYLE J.D. (1965) Hypernatremia complicating prolonged mannitol diuresis. *New. Eng. J. Med.* **272**, 1116

GOLD H., KWIT N.T., MESSELOFF C.R., KRAMER M.L., GOLFINS A.J., GREINER T.H., GOESSEL E.A., HUGHES J.H. and WARSHAU L. (1960) Comparison of chlorothiazide and of meralluride. New rapid method for quantitative evaluation of diuretics in bed-patients in congestive heart failure. *J. Amer. med. Ass.* **173,** 745

GOODOFF I.I. and MACBRIDE C.M. (1944) Heart failure in Addison's disease with myocardial changes of potassium deficiency. *J. clin. Endocrinol.* **4,** 30

★ GOODWIN J.F. (1958) The cardiographic assessment of electrolyte imbalance. *Proc. Roy. Soc. Med.* **51,** 801

GOODWIN J.F. and OAKLEY C.M. (1965) Potassium chloride and intestinal ulceration. *Lancet* **2,** 130

GORDILLO G., SOTO R.A., METCOFF J., LOPEZ E. and ANTILLON L.G. (1957) Intracellular composition and homeostatic mechanisms in severe chronic infantile malnutrition. *Pediatrics* **20,** 303

GORDON R.S. (1959) Exudative enteropathy. *Lancet* **1,** 325

GOTTSCHALK C.W. (1964) Osmotic concentration and dilution of the urine. *Amer. J. Med.* **36,** 670

GOULSTON K., HARRISON D.D. and SKYRING A.P. (1963) Effect of mineralocorticoids on the sodium/potassium ratio of human ileostomy fluid. *Lancet* **2,** 541

GOWENLOCK A.H., EMERY E.W. and BLACK D.A.K. (1960) Uptake of ^{42}K in the human fore-arm. *Clin. Sci.* **19,** 425

GOWENLOCK A.H. and WRONG O. (1962) Hyperaldosteronism secondary to renal ischaemia. *Quart. J. Med.* **31,** 323

GREENBERG E., DIVERTIE M.B. and WOOLNER L.B. (1964) A review of unused systemic manifestations associated with carcinoma. *Amer. J. Med.* **36,** 106

GREENOUGH W.B., SONNENBLICK E.H., JANUSZEWICZ V. and LARAGH J.H. (1962) Correction of hyperaldosteronism and of massive fluid retention of unknown cause by sympathomimetic agents. *Amer. J. Med.* **33,** 603

GREENMAN L., SHALER J.B. and DANOWSKI T.S. (1953) Biochemical disturbances and clinical symptoms during prolonged exchange resin therapy in congestive heart failure. *Amer. J. Med.* **14,** 391

GROSS E.G., DEXTER J.D. and ROTH R.G. (1966) Hypokalemic myopathy with myoglobinuria associated with licorice ingestion. *New Eng. J. Med.* **274,** 602

GRUMER H.A., DERRYBERRY W., DUBIN A. and WALDSTEIN S.S. (1962) Idiopathic, episodic inappropriate secretion of antiuretic hormone. *Amer. J. Med.* **32,** 954

GULYASSY P.F., STRIHOU C.Y. and SCHWARTZ W.B. (1962) On the mechanism of nitrate-induced alkalosis. The possible role of selective chloride depletion in acid-base regulation. *J. clin. Invest.* **41,** 1850

★ HAJDU S. and LEONARD E. (1959) The cellular basis of cardiac glycoside action. *Pharmacol. Rev.* **11,** 173

HAMWI G.J. and URBACH S. (1953) Body compartments, their measurement and application to clinical medicine. *Metabolism* **2,** 391

HARDT L.L. and RIVERS A.B. (1923) Toxic manifestations following the alkaline treatment of peptic ulcer. *Arch. intern. Med.* **31,** 171

HARRISON H.E., DARROW D.C. and YANNET H. (1936) Total electrolyte content of animals and its probable relation to distribution of body water. *J. Biol. Chem.,* **113,** 515

HARRISON H.E. and FINBERG L. (1959) Hypernatremic dehydration. *Pediat. Clin. N. Amer.* **6,** 193

HARRISON H.E., TOMPSETT R.R. and BARR D.P. (1943) The serum potassium in two cases of sprue. *Proc. Soc. Exp. Biol., N.Y.* **54,** 314

HARRIS E.A., JULIAN D.G. and OLIVER M.F. (1960) Atrial tachycardia with atrioventricular block due to digitalis poisoning. *Brit. med. J.* **2,** 1409

HARTMANN R.C. and MELLINKOFF S.M. (1955) Relationships of platelets to serum potassium concentration. *J. clin. Invest.* **34,** 938

HAYS R.M., McHUGH P.R. and WILLIAMS H.E. (1963) Absence of thirst in association with hydrocephalus. *New Eng. J. Med.* **269,** 227

HECKMAN B.A. and WALSH J.H. (1967) Hypernatremia complicating sodium sulfate therapy for hypercalcemic crisis. *New Eng. J. Med.* **276,** 1082

HELLMAN D.E., AU W.Y.W. and BARTTER F.C. (1965) Evidence for a direct effect of parathyroid hormone on urinary acidification. *Amer. J. Physiol.* **209,** 643

HERMAN R.H. and McDOWELL M.K. (1963) Hyperkalemic paralysis (adynamia episodica hereditaria) *Amer. J. Med.* **35,** 749

HIATT R.B. (1951) The pathologic physiology of congenital megacolon. *Ann. Surg.* **133,** 313

* HILLS A.G. (1959) Selective hypoaldosteronism. *Amer. J. Med.* **26,** 503

HIERHOLZER K. (1961) Secretion of potassium and acidification in collecting ducts of mammalian kidney. *Amer. J. Physiol.* **201,** 318

HOLLIDAY M.A. (1955) Acute metabolic alkalosis: its effect on potassium and acid excretion. *J. clin. Invest.* **34,** 428

HOWARD P., DUFF R.S., OWEN G. and BAKER W.T. (1963) Observations on capillary permeability in acute pancreatitis. *Lancet* **2,** 707

HUCKABEE W.E. (1961) Abnormal resting blood lactate. II. Lactate acidosis. *Amer. J. Med.* **30,** 840

HUDSON J.B., CHOBANIAN A.V. and RELMAN A.S. (1957) Hypoaldosteronism. A clinical study of a patient with an isolated adrenal mineralocorticoid deficiency, resulting in hyperkalemia and Stokes-Adams attacks. *New Engl. J. Med.* **257,** 529

HUNT J.N. (1956) The influence of dietary sulphur on the urinary output of acid in man. *Clin. Sci.* **15,** 119

HURST P.E., MORRISON R.B.I., TIMONER J., METCALFE-GIBSON A. and WRONG O. (1963) The effect of oral anion exchange resins on faecal anions. Comparison with calcium salts and aluminium hydroxide. *Clin. Sci.* **24,** 187

IRVINE R.O.H., SAUNDERS S.J., MILNE M.D. and CRAWFORD M.A. (1961) Gradients of potassium and hydrogen ion in potassium-deficient voluntary muscle. *Clin. Sci.* **20,** 1

JENKINS J.S. (1961) Progesterone and norethisterone in cyclical oedema and ascites. *Brit. med. J.* **2,** 861

JONES E.S. and SACHIARI G. (1963) Method for providing metabolic balance during intensive patient-care. *Lancet* **2,** 19

JONES E. SHERWOOD and PEASTON M.J.T. (1966) Metabolic care during acute illnesses. *Practitioner.* **196,** 271

JONES J.H. and PETERS D.K. (1966) Measurement of capillary permeability to plasma proteins by a gel-filtration technique. *Clin. Sci.* **31,** 389

JONES N.F. and MILLS I.H. (1964) Reversible renal potassium loss with urinary tract infection. *Amer. J. Med.* **37,** 305

JONES R.V., McSWINEY R.R. and BROOKS R.V. (1959) Periodic paralysis. Sodium metabolism and aldosterone output in two cases. *Lancet,* **1,** 177

JOSEPHSON B. (1961) *Chemistry and Therapy of Electrolyte Disorders.* Springfield, Ill., 1961

KASSIRER J.P., BERKMAN P.M., LAWRENZ D.R. and SCHWARTZ W.B. (1965) The critical role of chloride in the correction of hypokalemic alkalosis in man. *Amer. J. Med.* **38,** 172

KAYE M. (1966) An investigation into the cause of hyponatremia in the syndrome of inappropriate secretion of antidiuretic hormone. *Amer. J. Med.* **41,** 910

KEATING R.E., WEICHSELBAUM T.E., ALANIS M., MARGRAF H.W. and ELMAN R. (1953) The movement of potassium during experimental acidosis and alkalosis in the nephrectomized dog. *Surg. Gynecol. Obstet.* **96,** 323

KENNEDY Q.C., LINTON A.L., LUKE R.G. and RENFREW S. (1963) Electroencephalographic changes during haemodialysis. *Lancet* **1,** 408

KERPEL-FRONIUS E. (1935) Über die Beziehungen zwischen Salz- und Wasserhaushalt bei experimentellen Wasserverlüsten. *Z. Kinderheilk.* **57,** 489

KEYE J.D. (1952) Death in potassium deficiency; report of a case including morphologic findings. *Circulation* **5,** 766

KLEEMAN C.R., HEWITT W.L. and GUZE L.B. (1960) Pyelonephritis. *Medicine, Baltimore* **39,** 3

KLEEMAN C.R. and MAXWELL M.H. (1959) Contributing role of extrarenal factors in the polyuria of potassium depletion. *New Eng. J. Med.* **260,** 268

★ KOEFOED-JOHNSON V. and USSING H.H. (1960) Ion transport. In *Mineral Metabolism,* ed. C.L. Comar and F. Bronner. New York, 1960

KREBS H.A. (1954) Excursion into the borderland of biochemistry and philosophy. *Bull. Johns Hopk. Hosp.,* **95,** 45

KÜHNS K. (1954) Die Herztätigkeit bei Störungen des Kaliumstoffwechsels durch Kochsalz- und Na-PAS-Infusionen. *Verh. Dtsch. Ges. Kreisl. Forsch.* **20,** 389

KUNIN A.S., SURAWICZ B. and SIMS E.A.H. (1962) Decrease in serum potassium concentrations and appearance of cardiac arrhythmias during infusion of potassium with glucose in potassium-depleted patients. *New Eng. J. Med.* **266,** 228

LADELL W.S.S., WATERLOW J.C. and HUDSON M.F. (1944) Desert climate. Physiological and clinical observations. *Lancet* **2,** 491 and 527

LANCET (1965) Annotation—Respiratory acidosis in bronchial asthma. *Lancet* **2,** 632

LANDERMAN N.S., WEBSTER M.E., BECKER E.L. and RATCLIFFE H.E. (1962) Hereditary angioneurotic edema. II. Deficiency of inhibitor for serum globulin permeability factor and/or plasma kallikrein. *J. Allergy.* **33,** 330

LANGGÅRD H. and SMITH W.O. (1962) Self-induced water intoxication without predisposing illness. *New Eng. J. Med.* **266**, 378

LANT A.F. and WILSON G.M. (1967) Diuretics. Chapter in *Renal Diseases* (2nd edn.), ed. D.A.K. Black. Oxford, 1967

LARAGH J.H. (1954) The effect of potassium chloride on hyponatremia. *J. clin. Invest.* **33**, 807

LARAGH J.H. (1962) Hormones and the pathogenesis of congestive heart failure: vasopressin, aldosterone and angiotensin II. *Circulation*, **25**, 1015

LARAGH J.H., CANNON P.J., BENTZEL C.J., SICINSKI A.M. and MELTZER J.I. (1963) Angiotensin II, norepinephrine, and renal transport of electrolytes and water in normal man and in cirrhosis with ascites. *J. clin. Invest.* **42**, 1179

★ LEAF A. (1962) The clinical and physiologic significance of the serum sodium concentration. *New Eng. J. Med.* **267**, 24

LEAF A. and CAMARA A.A. (1949) Renal tubular secretion of potassium in man. *J. Amer. med. Ass.* **155**, 1204

LEDINGHAM I.McA. and NORMAN J.N. (1962) Acid-base studies in experimental cardiac arrest. *Lancet* **2**, 967

LEHMANN J.E. (1937) The effect of changes in the potassium-calcium balance on the action of mammalian A nerve fibres. *Amer. J. Physiol.* **118**, 613

LEITHEAD C.S. and LIND A.R. (1964) *Heat stress and heat disorders.* London, 1964

LEMANN J., LITZOW J.R. and LENNON E.J. (1966) The effects of chronic acid loads in normal man: Further evidence for the participation of bone mineral in the defence against chronic metabolic acidosis. *J. clin. Invest.* **45**, 1608

LEQUESNE L.P. and LEWIS A.A.G. (1953) Postoperative retention of water and sodium. *Lancet* **1**, 153

LE VEEN H.H., PASTERNACK H.S., LUSTRIN I., SHAPIRO R.B., BECKER E. and HELFT A.E. (1960) Hemorrhage and transfusion as the major cause of cardiac arrest. *J. Amer. med. Ass.* **173**, 770

LEVER A.F. (1965) The vasa recta and counter-current multiplication. *Acta med. Scand.*, Supp. **434**, 1

LEVINSKY N.G. (1966) Management of emergencies—hyperkalemia. *New Eng. J. Med.* **274**, 1076

LEWIS B.I. (1954) Chronic hyperventilation syndrome. *J. Amer. med. Ass.* **155**, 1204

LINDEMAN R.D., VAN BUREN H.C. and RAISZ L.G. (1961) Effect of steroids on water diuresis and vasopressin sensitivity. *J. clin. Invest.* **40**, 152

LING G.N. (1952) The role of phosphate in the maintenance of the resting potential and selective ionic accumulation in frog muscle cells. *Phosphorus Metabolism— a Symposium.* **2**, 748. Baltimore, 1952

LITCHFIELD J.A. (1959) Low-potassium syndrome resulting from the use of purgative drugs. *Gastroenterol.* **37**, 483

LITCHFIELD J.A. and GADDIE R. (1958) The measurement of the phase distribution of water and electrolytes in skeletal muscle by the analysis of small samples. *Clin. Sci.* **17**, 483

LLAURADO J.G. and WOODRUFF M.F.A. (1957) Postoperative transient aldosteronism. *Surgery*, **42,** 313

LOCKEY E., LONGMORE D.B., ROSS D.N. and STURRIDGE M.F. (1966) Potassium and open-heart surgery. *Lancet* **1,** 671

LOEB R.F. (1941–42) Adrenal cortex and electrolyte behaviour. *Harvey Lect.* **37,** 100

LOWE K.G. (1953) Metabolic studies with protein-free, electrolyte-free diet in man. *Clin. Sci.* **12,** 57

LOWE K.G., STOWERS J.M. and WALKER W.F. (1959) Electrolyte disturbances in patients with uretero-sigmoidostomy. *Scot. med. J.* **4,** 473

LOWN B. and LEVINE H.D. (1958) *Atrial Arrhythmias, Digitalis, and Potassium.* New York, 1958

LUBRAN M. and McALLEN P.M. (1951) Potassium deficiency in ulcerative colitis. *Quart. J. Med.* **20,** 221

LUKE R.G. and LEVITIN H. (1967) Impaired renal conservation of chloride and the acid-base changes associated with potassium-depletion in the rat. *Clin. Sci.* **32,** 511

MACALLUM A.B. (1926) The paleochemistry of the body fluids and tissues. *Physiol. Rev.* **6,** 316

MACKENZIE G.J., FLENLEY D.C., TAYLOR S.H., McDONALD A.H., STAUNTON H.P. and DONALD K.W. (1964) Circulatory and respiratory studies in myocardial infarction and cardiogenic shock. *Lancet* **2,** 825

McCANCE R.A. (1936) Medical problems in mineral metabolism. *Lancet* **1,** 823

★ McCANCE R.A. (1950) Renal physiology in infancy. *Amer. J. Med.* **9,** 229

★ McCANCE R.A. (1953) Overnutrition and undernutrition. *Lancet* **2,** 685 and 739

McCANCE R.A. and WIDDOWSON E.N. (1951) Composition of the body. *Brit. med. Bull.* **7,** 297; and A method of breaking down the body weights of living persons into terms of extracellular fluid, cell mass and fat, and some applications of it to physiology and medicine. *Proc. Roy. Soc. B.*, **138,** 115

McCRACKEN B.H. and PARSONS F.M. (1958) Use of Nilevar (17-ethyl-19-nortestosterone) to suppress protein catabolism in acute renal failure. *Lancet* **2,** 855

McFARLAND L.Z. (1964) Minimal salt load required to induce secretion from the nasal salt-glands of sea gulls. *Nature, Lond.* **204,** 202

MACH R., FABRE J., MULLER A., NEHER A. and BORTH R. (1955) Oedème idiopathique par rétention sodique avec hyperaldostéronurie. *Bull. Mém. Soc. Hôp. Paris*, 1955, p. 726

MAHLER R.F. and STANBURY S.W. (1956) Potassium-losing renal disease. *Quart. J. Med.* **25,** 21

MALAMUD N., HAYMAKER W. and CUSTER R.P. (1946) Heat stroke: clinico-pathologic study of 125 fatal cases. *Milit. Surg.* **99,** 397

MANERY J.F. (1954) Water and electrolyte metabolism. *Physiol Rev.* **34,** 334

MANITIUS A., LEVITIN H., BECK D. and EPSTEIN F.H. (1960) On the mechanism of impairment of renal concentrating ability in potassium deficiency. *J. clin. Invest.* **39,** 684

MAREN T.H., SORSDAHL O.A. and DICKHAUS A.J. (1961) Renal action of acetazol-amide in extracellular alkalosis of potassium deficiency. *Amer. J. Physiol.* **200**, 170

MARRIOTT H.J.L. (1953) Iatrogenic salt depletion. *Ann. intern. Med.* **39**, 152

MARRIOTT H.L. (1947) Water and salt depletion. *Brit. med. J.* **1**, 245, 285 and 328. (Revised edition, 1950. *Water and Salt Depletion*. Blackwell, Oxford, 1950)

Medical Research Council memorandum No. 26 (1952). *The Treatment of Acute Dehydration in Infants*. London, 1952

MELVIN K.E.W., FARRELLY R.O. and NORTH J.D.K. (1963) Ethacrynic acid: a new oral diuretic. *Brit. med. J.* **1**, 1521

MERRILL J.P. (1956) Electrolyte changes in renal failure. *Metabolism* **5**, 419

★ MERRILL J.P. (1962) Acute renal failure. Chapter 13 in *Renal Disease*, ed. D.A.K. Black. Blackwell, Oxford, 1962

METCOFF J., FRENK S., GORDILLO G., GÓMEZ F., RAMOS-GALVÁN R., CRAVIOTO J., JANEWAY C.A. and GAMBLE J.L. (1957) Intracellular composition and homeo-static mechanisms in severe chronic infantile malnutrition. *Pediatrics* **20**, 317

MILLER R.B., TYSON I. and RELMAN A.S. (1963) pH of isolated resting skeletal muscle and its relation to potassium content. *Amer. J. Physiol.* **204**, 1048

★ MILNE M.D., SCRIBNER B.H. and CRAWFORD M.A. (1958) Non-ionic diffusion and the excretion of weak acids and bases. *Amer. J. Med.* **24**, 709

MILNE M.D., STANBURY S.W. and THOMSON A.E. (1952) Observations on the Fanconi syndrome and renal hyperchloraemic acidosis in the adult. *Quart. J. Med.* **21**, 61

★ MILLS J.N. (1966) Human circadian rhythms. *Physiol. Rev.* **46**, 128

MILLS J.N., THOMAS S. and WILLIAMSON K.S. (1960) The acute effect of hydro-cortisone, deoxycorticosterone, and aldosterone upon the excretion of sodium, potassium and acid by the human kidney. *J. Physiol.* **151**, 312

MILLS J.N., THOMAS S. and WILLIAMSON K.S. (1962) The extent of the adrenal influence upon renal electrolyte excretion in the healthy man on a normal diet, and its contribution to the renal changes on standing. *J. Endocrinol.* **23**, 365

MINOT A.S., DODD K. and SAUNDERS J.M. (1934) The acidosis of guanidine intoxi-cation. *J. clin. Invest.* **13**, 917

MITTRA B. (1965) Potassium, glucose and insulin in the treatment of myocardial infarction. *Lancet* **2**, 607

MIZGALA H.F., LASSER R.P. and FRIEDBERG C.K. (1963) The treatment of refractory retention of fluid with oral L-arginine monohydrochloride and meralluride. *Amer. Heart J.* **65**, 5

MOHAMED S.D., CHAPMAN R.S. and CROOKS J. (1966) Hypokalaemia, flaccid quad-ruparesis, and myoglobinuria with carbenoxolone (Biogastrone). *Brit. med. J.* **1**, 1581

MOLHUYSEN J.A., GERBRANDY J., DE VRIES L.A., DE JONG J.C., LENSTRA J.B., TURNER K.P. and BORST J.G.G. (1950) A liquorice extract with deoxycortone-like action. *Lancet* **2**, 381

M

MOLMAR Z., LARSEN K. and SPARGO B. (1962) Heart lesions due to potassium depletion. *Arch. Path.* **74,** 339

MONCRIEFF A. (1960) Biochemistry of mental defect. *Lancet* **2,** 273

MOORE F.D. (1954) The low sodium syndromes of surgery. *J. Amer. med. Ass.* **154,** 379

MOORE F.D. (1963) Tris buffer, mannitol, and low-viscous Dextran: three new solutions for old problems. *Surg. Clin. N. Amer.* **43,** 577

MOORE F.D. and BALL M.R. (1952) *The Metabolic Response to Surgery.* Springfield, 1952

MOORE F.D., BOLING E.A., DITMORE H.B., SICULAR A., TETERICK, J.E., ELLISON A.E., HOYE S.J. and BALL M.R. (1955) Body sodium and potassium. V. The relationship of alkalosis, potassium deficiency and surgical stress to acute hypokalemia in man. *Metabolism* **4,** 379

MOORE F.D., EDELMAN I.S., OLNEY J.M., JAMES A.H., BROOKS L. and WILSON G.M. (1954) Body sodium and potassium. III. Interrelated trends in alimentary, renal, and cardio-vascular disease; lack of correlation between body stores and plasma concentration. *Metabolism* **4,** 334

MOORE F.D., HALEY H.B., BERING E.A., BROOKS L. and EDELMAN I.S. (1952) Further observations on total body-water. II. Changes of body composition in disease. *Surg. Gynecol., Obstet.* **95,** 155

MORRISON A.B., RAWSON A.J. and FITTS W.T. (1962) The syndrome of refractory watery diarrhoea and hypokalaemia in patients with a non-insulin-secreting islet-cell tumour. *Amer. J. Med.* **32,** 119

MOYER J.H. and FUCHS M. (1960) *Edema: Mechanisms and Management.* Philadelphia, 1960

MUDGE G.H. (1953) Potassium imbalance. *Bull. N.Y. Acad. Med.* **29,** 846

MULROW P.J. and GANONG W.F. (1961) The effect of hemorrhage upon aldosterone secretion in normal and hypophysectomized dogs. *J. clin. Invest.* **40,** 579

MUNRO D.S. (1959) The measurement of 'spaces'—methods and significance. Chapter 3 in *Clinical effects of Electrolyte Disturbances,* ed. E.J. Ross. London, 1959

MYHRE L.G. and KESSLER W.V. (1966) Body density and potassium 40 measurements of body composition as related to age. *J. Appl. Physiol.* **21,** 1251

NABARRO J.D.N., SPENCER A.G. and STOWERS J.M. (1952) Metabolic studies in severe diabetic ketosis. *Quart. J. Med.* **21,** 225

NADAL J.W., PEDERSON S. and MADDOCK W.G. (1941) Comparison between dehydration from salt loss and from water deprivation. *J. clin. Invest.* **20,** 691

NAHAS G.G. (1966) [Editor] Current concepts of acid-base measurement. *Ann. N.Y. Acad. Sci.* **133,** 1

★ NATIONAL RESEARCH COUNCIL publication (1954). Sodium restricted diets: the rationale, complications, and practical aspects of their use. *National Research Council Publication* 325, Washington. (Summary in *J. Amer. Med. Ass.* **156,** 1081, 1171 and 1252)

NEAVERSON M.A. (1966) Metabolic acidosis in acute myocardial infarction. *Brit. med. J.* **2**, 383

NEEDLE M.A., KALOYANIDES G.J. and SCHWARTZ W.B. (1964) The effects of selective depletion of hydrochloric acid on acid-base and electrolyte equilibrium. *J. clin. Invest.* **43**, 1836

NELSON W.P., ROSENBAUM J.D. and STRAUSS M.B. (1951) Hyponatremia in hepatic cirrhosis following paracentesis. *J. clin. Invest.* **30**, 738

NEWBURGH L.H. and JOHNSTON M.W. (1942) The insensible loss of water. *Physiol. Rev.* **22**, 1

NEYZI M., BAILEY M. and TALBOT N.B. (1958) Effects of varying infusion time on maintenance fluid therapy. *New Eng. J. Med.* **258**, 1239

NICHOLS G., NICHOLS N., WEIL W.B. and WALLACE W.M. (1953) The direct measurement of the extracellular phase of tissues. *J. clin. Invest.* **32**, 1299

NOBLE M.I.M., TRENCHARD D. and GUZ A. (1966) The value of diuretics in respiratory failure. *Lancet* **2**, 257

OLEESKY S. and STANBURY S.W. (1951) Effect of oral cortisone on water excretion in Addison's disease and hypopituitarism. *Lancet* **2**, 664

OLIVER J., MACDOWELL M., WELT L.G., HOLLIDAY M.A., HOLLANDER W., WINTERS R.W., WILLIAMS T.F. and SEGAR W.E. (1957) The renal lesions of electrolyte imbalance. I. The structural alterations in potassium-depleted rats. *J. exp. Med.* **106**, 563

ORAM S., RESNEKOV L. and DAVIES P. (1960) Digitalis as a cause of paroxysmal atrial tachycardia with atrio-ventricular block. *Brit. med. J.* **2**, 1402

ORLOFF J. and BURG M.B. (1963) Vasopressin-resistant diabetes insipidus. Chapter 34 in *Diseases of the Kidney*, ed. M.B. Strauss and L.G. Welt. Boston, 1963

OWEN J.A., DUDLEY H.A.F. and MASTERTON J.P. (1965) Acid-base status assessed from measurements of hydrogen-ion concentration and P_{CO_2}. *Lancet* **2**, 660

PAK POY R.K. and WRONG O. (1960) The urinary P_{CO_2} in renal disease. *Clin. Sci.* **19**, 631

PAPPENHEIMER J.R. (1965) The ionic composition of cerebral extracellular fluid and its relation to control of breathing. *Harvey Lect.* **61**, 71

PARSONS F.M. and FORE H. (1963) High carbohydrate intake for oral use in acute renal failure. *Lancet* **2**, 386

PEARSE A.G.E. and MACPHERSON C.R. (1958) Renal histochemistry in potassium depletion. *J. Path. Bact.* **75**, 69

PEARSON R.G. (1966) Acids and bases. *Science* **63**, 873

PERKINS J.G., PETERSEN A.B. and RILEY J.A. (1950) Renal and cardiac lesions in potassium deficiency due to chronic diarrhoea. *Amer. J. Med.* **8**, 115

PHILLIPS R.A. (1966) Cholera in the perspective of 1966. *Ann. intern. Med.* **65**, 922

PITTMAN J.G. (1963) Water intoxication due to oxytocin. *New Eng. J. Med.* **268**, 481

* PITTS R.F. (1959) *The Physiological Basis of Diuretic Therapy.* Thomas, Springfield, 1959

* PITTS R.F. (1963) *Physiology of the Kidney and Body Fluids.* Year Book, Chicago, 1963

PITTS R.F. and DUGGAN J.J. (1950) Studies on diuretics. II. The relationship between glomerular filtration rate, proximal tubular absorption of sodium, and diuretic efficacy of mercurials. *J. clin. Invest.* **29,** 372

PLATT R. (1950) Sodium and potassium excretion in chronic renal failure. *Clin. Sci.* **9,** 367

PLATT R. (1952) Structural and functional adaptation in renal failure. *Brit. med. J.* **1,** 1313

PLATT R. (1959) Some consequences of renal inadequacy. *Lancet* **1,** 159

PLATTS M.M. (1966) Electrolyte excretion in uraemia. *Clin. Sci.* **30,** 453

PLATTS M.M. and GREAVES M.S. (1957) The composition of the blood in respiratory acidosis. *Clin. Sci.* **16,** 695

POLLEN R.H. and WILLIAMS R.H. (1960) Hyperkalemic neuromyopathy in Addison's disease. *New Eng. J. Med.* **263,** 273

POSNER J.B. and JACOBS D.R. (1964) Isolated analdosteronism. I. Clinical entity, with manifestations of persistent hyperkalemia, periodic paralysis, salt-losing tendency, and acidosis. *Metabolism* **13,** 513

PREEDY J.R.K. and RICHARDSON J.E. (1956). Control of water and electrolyte disorders. A simple chart. *Lancet* **1,** 223

PRENTICE T.C., SIRI W., BERLIN N.I., HYDE G.M., PARSONS R.J., JOINER E.E. and LAWRENCE J.H. (1952) Studies of total body water with tritium. *J. clin. Invest.* **31,** 412

PRESHAW R.M. and HARVEY P.W.C. (1963) Post-operative hypotension due to paroxysmal atrial tachycardia with block. *Brit. med. J.* **2,** 152

RECTOR F.C., BLOOMER H.A. and SELDIN D.W. (1964) Effect of potassium deficiency on the reabsorption of bicarbonate in the proximal tubule of the rat kidney. *J. clin. Invest.* **43,** 1976

RECTOR F.C., BRUNNER F.P. and SELDIN D.W. (1966) Mechanisms of glomerulotubular balance. I. *J. clin. Invest.* **45,** 590

RECTOR F.C., SELDIN D.W., ROBERTS A.D. and SMITH J.S. (1960) The role of plasma CO_2 tension and carbonic anhydrase activity in the renal reabsorption of bicarbonate. *J. clin. Invest.* **39,** 1706

REFSUM H.E. (1961) Hypokalemic alkalosis with paradoxical aciduria during artificial ventilation of patients with pulmonary insufficiency and high plasma bicarbonate concentration. *Scand. J. Clin. Lab. Invest.* **13,** 481

REICHSTEIN T.S., SIMPSON S.A., TAIT J.F., WETTSTEIN A., NEHER R. and v. EUW J. (1953) Isolation from adrenal of a new crystalline hormone with especial high effectiveness on mineral metabolism. *Experientia* **9,** 333

REID H.A. (1961) Myoglobinuria and sea-snake-bite poisoning. *Brit. med. J.* **1,** 1284

REIMER A., SCHOCK H.A. and NEWBURGH L.H. (1951) Certain aspects of potassium metabolism. *J. Amer. Dietet. Ass.* **29,** 1042

RELMAN A.S. (1964) Renal acidosis and renal excretion of acid in health and disease. *Adv. intern. Med.* **12,** 295

RELMAN A.S., LENNON E.J. and LEMANN J. (1961) Endogenous production of fixed acid and the measurement of the net balance of acid in normal subjects. *J. clin. Invest.* **40**, 1621

RELMAN A.S. and SCHWARTZ W.B. (1955) The nephropathy of potassium depletion. A clinico-pathologic entity. *J. clin. Invest.* **34**, 959

RELMAN A.S. and SCHWARTZ W.B. (1967) Effects of electrolyte disorders on renal structure and function. Chapter in *Renal Disease*, ed. D.A.K. Black. Blackwell, Oxford, 1967

RINGER S. (1883) A further contribution regarding the influence of the different constituents of the blood on the contraction of the heart. *J. Physiol.* **4**, 29

ROBERTS K.E., RANDALL H.T., PHILBIN P. and LIPTON R. (1954) Changes in extracellular water and electrolytes and the renal compensations in chronic alkalosis, as compared to those occurring in acute alkalosis. *Surgery* **36**, 599

ROBERTS K.E., RANDALL H.T., VANAMEE P. and POPPELL J.W. (1956) Renal mechanisms involved in bicarbonate reabsorption. *Metabolism* **5**, 404

ROBIN E.D. (1963) Abnormalities of acid-base regulation in chronic pulmonary disease, with special reference to hypercapnia and extracellular alkalosis. *New Eng. J. Med.* **268**, 917

ROBIN E.D., DAVIS R.P. and REES S.B. (1959) Salicylate intoxication with special reference to the development of hypokalemia. *Amer. J. Med.* **26**, 869

* ROBINSON J.R. (1965) *Fundamentals of Acid-Base Regulation*, 2nd edn. Blackwell, Oxford, 1965.

ROBINSON J.R. and McCANCE R.A. (1952) Water metabolism. *Ann. Rev. Physiol.* **14**, 115

ROSENHEIM M.L. and SPENCER A.G. (1956) Treatment of nephrotic syndrome with cation-exchange resins and high-protein low-sodium diet. *Lancet* **2**, 313

ROSS E.J., CRABBÉ J., RENOLD A.E., EMERSON K. and THORN G.W. (1958) A case of massive edema in association with an aldosterone-secreting adrenocortical adenoma. *Amer. J. Med.* **25**, 278

ROUSSAK N.J. (1952) Fatal hypokalemic alkalosis with tetany during liquorice and PAS therapy. *Brit. med. J.* **1**, 360

ROWNTREE L.G. (1922) The water balance of the body. *Physiol. Rev.* **2**, 116

ROY A.D. and ELLIS H. (1959) Potassium-secreting tumours of the large intestine. *Lancet* **1**, 759

SALTZMAN H.A., HEYMAN A. and SIEKER H.O. (1963) Correlation of clinical and physiologic manifestations of sustained hyperventilation. *New Eng. J. Med.* **268**, 1131

SANDERSON P.H. (1967) Renal potassium wasting in hypercalcaemia. *Brit. med. J.* **1**, 679

SANTOS R.F. (1959) Extrarenal action of adrenal glands on potassium metabolism. *Amer. J. Physiol.* **197**, 643

SAPIR D.G., LEVINE D.Z. and SCHWARTZ W.B. (1967) The effects of chronic hypoxemia on electrolyte and acid-base equilibrium: an examination of normocapnic hypoxemia and of the influence of hypoxemia on the adaptation to chronic hypercapnia. *J. clin. Invest.* **46**, 369

SCHMIDT-NIELSEN B. and SLADEN W.J.L. (1958) Nasal salt secretion in the Humboldt penguin. *Nature, Lond.* **181**, 1217

SCHOTTSTAEDT W.W., PINSKY R.H., MACKLER D. and WOLF S. (1958) Sociologic, psychologic, and metabolic observations on patients in the community of a metabolic ward. *Amer. J. Med.* **25**, 248

SCHREINER G.E. (1967) Acute renal failure. Chapter in *Renal Disease* (2nd edn.), ed. D.A.K. Black. Blackwell, Oxford, 1967

SCHROEDER H.A. (1949) Renal failure associated with low extracellular sodium chloride. *J. Amer. med. Ass.* **141**, 117

SCHWARTZ W.B., HALL P.W., HAYS R.M. and RELMAN A.S. (1959) On the mechanism of acidosis in chronic renal disease. *J. clin. Invest.* **38**, 39

SCHWARTZ W.B., HAYS R.M., POLAK A. and HAYNIE G.D. (1961) Effects of chronic hypercapnia on electrolyte and acid-base equilibrium. II. Recovery, with special reference to the influence of chloride intake. *J. clin. Invest.* **40**, 1238

SCHWARTZ W.B. and RELMAN A.S. (1953) Metabolic and renal studies in chronic potassium depletion resulting from overuse of laxatives. *J. clin. Invest.* **32**, 258

SCHWARTZ W.B. and RELMAN A.S. (1963) A critique of the parameters used in the evaluation of acid-base disorders: 'whole-blood buffer base' and 'standard bicarbonate' compared with blood pH and plasma bicarbonate concentration. *New Eng. J. Med.* **268**, 1382

SCHWARTZ W.B. and WALLACE W.M. (1951) Electrolyte equilibrium during mercurial diuresis. *J. clin. Invest.* **30**, 1089

SCHWARTZ W.B., TASSEL D. and BARTTER F.C. (1960) Further observations on hyponatremia and renal sodium loss probably resulting from inappropriate secretion of antidiuretic hormone. *New Eng. J. Med.* **262**, 743

SCHWARTZ W.B. and WATERS W.C. (1962) Lactate versus bicarbonate. A reconsideration of the therapy of metabolic acidosis. *Amer. J. Med.* **32**, 831

SCRIBNER B.H. (1958) Discussion on p. 269 of *Water and Electrolyte Metabolism in Relation to Age and Sex*, ed. Wolstenholme and O'Connor. London, 1958

SCRIBNER B.H. and BURNELL J.M. (1956) Interpretation of the serum potassium concentration. *Metabolism* **5**, 468

* SELKURT E.E. (1954) Sodium excretion by the mammalian kidney. *Physiol. Rev.* **34**, 287

SENSENIG D.M. and CAMPBELL R.E. (1957) Total gastrectomy with reference to chronic hypokalemia. *Ann. Surg.* **145**, 1119

SHALDON S., McLAREN J.R. and SHERLOCK S. (1960) Resistant ascites treated by combined diuretic therapy. *Lancet* **1**, 609

SHAKER Y. (1966) Thirst fever, with a characteristic temperature pattern, in infants in Kuwait. *Brit. med. J.* **1**, 586

SHAW A.B., BAZZARD F.J., BOOTH E.M., NILWARANGKUR S. and BERLYNE G.M. (1965) The treatment of chronic renal failure by a modified Giovannetti diet. *Quart. J. Med.* **34**, 237

SHAW D.M. (1966) Mineral metabolism, mania and melancholia. *Brit. med. J.* **2,** 262

SHERLOCK S. (1958) *Diseases of the Liver and Biliary System.* Blackwell, Oxford, 1958

SHIRES G.T. and HOLMAN J. (1948) Dilution acidosis. *Ann. intern. Med.* **28,** 557

SHNITKA T.K., FRIEDMAN M.H.W., KIDD E.G. and MACKENZIE W.C. (1961) Villous tumors of the rectum and colon characterized by severe fluid and electrolyte loss. *Surg. Gynecol. Obstet.* **112,** 609

SHOHL A.T. (1939) *Mineral Metabolism.* New York, 1939

SIMPSON H. and O'DUFFY J. (1967) Need for clarity in infant feeding instructions. *Brit. med. J.* **2,** 536

SIMPSON S.A., TAIT J.F. and BUSH I.E. (1952) Secretion of a salt-retaining hormone by the mammalian adrenal cortex. *Lancet* **2,** 226

SIMS E.A.H., WELT L.G., ORLOFF J. and NEEDHAM J.W. (1950) Asymptomatic hyponatremia in pulmonary tuberculosis. *J. clin. Invest.* **29,** 1545

SINGER R.B. and HASTINGS A.B. (1948) An improved clinical method for the estimation of disturbances of the acid-base balance of human blood. *Medicine, Baltimore* **27,** 223

SKANSE B. and HÖKFELT B. (1958) Hypoaldosteronism with otherwise intact adrenocortical function, resulting in a characteristic clinical entity. *Acta endocrinol.* **28,** 29

SKOU J.C. (1965) Enzymatic basis for active transport of Na^+ and K^+ across cell membrane. *Physiol. Rev.* **45,** 596

SLATON P.E. and BIGLIERI E.G. (1965) Hypertension and hyperaldosteronism of renal and adrenal origin. *Amer. J. Med.* **38,** 324

SMITH H.W. (1951) *The Kidney.* New York, 1951

* SMITH H.W. (1957) Salt and water volume receptors. An exercise in physiologic apologetics. *Amer. J. Med.* **23,** 623

SODEMAN W.A. (1960) Forward failure versus backward failure. P. 704 in *Edema*, ed. J.H. Moyer and M. Fuchs. Philadelphia, 1960

SOMLYO A.P. (1960) Molar sodium lactate antagonism of myocardial depressants. *Amer. Heart J.* **60,** 484

SPENCER A.G., ROSS E.J. and LLOYD-THOMAS H.G.L. (1954) Cation exchange in the gastro-intestinal tract. *Brit. med. J.* **1,** 603

STEWART J.S.S., STEWART W.K. and GILLIES H.G. (1962) Cardiac arrest and acidosis. *Lancet* **2,** 967

SUMMERSKILL W.H.J. (1960) Pathogenesis and treatment of disorders of water and electrolyte metabolism in hepatic disease. *Proc. Mayo Clin.* **35,** 89

SQUIRES R.D., HUTH E.J. and ELKINTON J.R. (1959) Experimental potassium depletion in normal human subjects. *J. clin. Invest.* **38,** 1134 and 1149

* STANBURY S.W. (1958) Some aspects of disordered renal tubular function. *Adv. intern. Med.* **9,** 231

STANBURY S.W. (1967) Bony complications of renal disease. Chapter in *Renal Disease*, ed. D.A.K. Black, Blackwell, Oxford 1967

STANBURY S.W. and MACAULAY D. (1957) Defects of renal tubular function in the nephrotic syndrome; observations on a nephrotic child with aminoaciduria, glycosuria, polyuria, tubular acidosis, and potassium depletion. *Quart. J. Med.* **26,** 7

STANBURY S.W. and THOMSON A.E. (1951) Diurnal variations in electrolyte excretion. *Clin. Sci.* **10,** 267

STANBURY S.W. and THOMSON A.E. (1952) Renal response to respiratory alkalosis. *Clin. Sci.* **11,** 357

STANBURY S.W. and MAHLER R.F. (1959) Salt-losing renal disease. *Quart. J. Med.* **28,** 425

STARLING E.H. (1909) *The Fluids of the Body.* London, 1909

STEWART J.S.S., MOSTERT J.W., HILTON D.D. and McGRATH D. (1965) Bicarbonate therapy during embolectomy. *Lancet* **2,** 1320

* STRAUSS M.B. (1957) *Body Water in Man.* London, 1957

STREETEN D.H.P. and VAUGHAN WILLIAMS E.M. (1952) Loss of cellular potassium as a cause of intestinal paralysis in dogs. *J. Physiol.* **118,** 149

STRONG J.A. (1951) Serum potassium deficiency during treatment with sodium P.A.S. and liquorice extract. *Brit. med. J.* **2,** 998

STUBBS J.D. and PENNYBACKER J. (1960) Reduction of intracranial pressure with hypertonic urea. *Lancet* **1,** 1094

SURAWICZ B., BRAUN H.A., CRUM W.B., KEMP R.L., WAGNER S. and BELLET S. (1957) Clinical manifestations of hypopotassemia. *Amer. J. med. Sci.* **233,** 603

SWALES J.D. (1964) Hypokalaemia and the electrocardiogram. *Lancet* **2,** 1365

TAIT J.F., BOUGAS J., LITTLE B., TAIT S.A.S. and FLOOD C. (1965) Splanchnic extraction and clearance of aldosterone in subjects with minimal and marked cardiac dysfunction. *J. clin. Endocrinol.* **25,** 219

TASHIMA C.K. (1965) Effect of prolonged hydrocortisone administration on potassium metabolism (letter). *Lancet* **1,** 866

TAYLOR W.H. (1962) Hypernatraemia in cerebral disorders. *J. clin. Path.* **15,** 211

THAYSEN J.H., LASSEN N.A. and MUNCK O. (1961) Sodium transport and oxygen consumption in the mammalian kidney. *Nature, Lond.* **190,** 919

THOMPSON G.S. and SHERWOOD JONES E. (1965) Errors in the measurement of serum electrolytes. *J. clin. Path.* **18,** 443

THOMSON A.E. (1957) Electrolyte studies in the respiratory paralysis of poliomyelitis. *Amer. J. Med.* **22,** 549

THREEFOOT S.A. (1962) Some factors influencing interpretation of studies of body water and electrolyte with isotopic tracers. *Progr. Cardiovasc. Dis.* **5,** 32

THORN G.W., KOEPF G.F. and CLINTON M. (1944) Renal failure simulating adrenocortical insufficiency. *New Eng. J. Med.* **231,** 76

THORN G.W., NELSON K.R. and THORN D.W. (1938) Study of mechanism of edema associated with menstruation. *Endocrinol.* **22,** 155

THURAU K. and SCHNEEMAN J. (1965) Die Natriumkonzentration an den Macula densa-Zellen als regulierender Faktor für des GlomerulumFilträt (Mikropunktions-versuche). *Klin. Wschr.* **43,** 410

TIMONER J., RIDDELL A.G. and CARR G.R. (1959) The effect of blood transfusion on the metabolic response to gastric surgery. *Clin. Sci.* **18**, 561

TINCKLER L.F. (1966) Fluid and electrolyte observations in tropical surgical practice. *Brit. med. J.* **1**, 1263

TYLER F.H., STEPHENS F.E., GUNN F.D. and PERKOFF G.T. (1951) Clinical manifestations and inheritance of a type of periodic paralysis without hypopotassaemia. *J. clin. Invest.* **30**, 492

URIST M.R. (1962) The bone—body-fluid continuum: calcium and phosphorus in the skeleton and blood of extinct and living vertebrates. *Perspectives Biol. Med.* **6**, 75

★ VANDER WERF C.A. (1961) *Acids, Bases, and the Chemistry of the Covalent Bond.* Reinhold, New York, 1961

VAN GOIDSENHOVEN G.M.-T., GRAY O.V., PRICE A.V. and SANDERSON P.H. (1954). The effect of prolonged administration of large doses of sodium bicarbonate in man. *Clin. Sci.* **13**, 383

VAN'T HOFF W. (1962) Familial myotonic periodic paralysis. *Quart. J. Med.* **31**, 385

VAN YPERSELE DE STRIHOU C., BRASSEUR L. and DE CONINCK J. (1966) The 'carbon dioxide response curve' for chronic hypercapnia in man. *New Eng. J. Med.* **275**, 117

VERE D.W. and KING C.E. (1960) The reaction to subcutaneous drainage in anasarca. *Lancet* **1**, 779

VERNEY E.P. (1947) Antidiuretic hormone and the factors which determine its release. *Proc. Roy. Soc. B.* **135**, 25

VERNEY E.B. (1948) Agents determining and influencing the functions of the pars nervosa of the pituitary. *Brit. med. J.* **2**, 119

WAKIM K.G. (1967) Reassessment of the source, mode and locus of action of antidiuretic hormone. *Amer. J. Med.* **42**, 394

WALKER W.G., JOST L.J., JOHNSON J.R. and KOWARSKI A. (1965) Metabolic observations on salt wasting in a patient with renal disease. *Amer. J. Med.* **39**, 505

WANGENSTEEN O.H. (1942) *Intestinal Obstructions*, 2nd edn. Springfield, 1952

WARD D.J. (1963) Fatal hypernatraemia after a saline emetic. *Brit. med. J.* **2**, 432

WARREN J.V. and STEAD E.A. (1944) The protein content of edema fluid in patients with acute glomerulonephritis. *Amer. J. med. Sci.* **208**, 618

WATTEN R.H., MORGAN F.M., SONGKHLA Y.N., VANIKIATI B. and PHILLIPS R.A. (1959) Water and electrolyte studies in cholera. *J. clin. Invest.* **38**, 1879

WEINBREN I. (1963) Spontaneous periodic oedema. A new syndrome. *Lancet* **2**, 544

WEISBERG H.F. (1962) *Water, Electrolyte and Acid-Base Balance*, 2nd edn. Baltimore, 1962

WELLS C.L., MORAN T.J. and COOPER W.M. (1962) Villous tumors of the rectosigmoid colon with severe electrolyte imbalance. *Amer. J. clin. Path.* **37**, 507

★ WELT L.G., HOLLANDER W. and BLYTHE W.B. (1960) The consequences of potassium depletion. *J. chron. Dis.* **11**, 213

WIDDOWSON E.M. and DICKERSON J.W.T. (1964) Chemical composition of the body. In *Mineral Metabolism*, Vol. II, Part A. Ed. C.L. Comar and F. Bronner. New York and London, 1964

WIDDOWSON E.M. and McCANCE R.A. (1956) The effect of development on the composition of the serum and extracellular fluids. *Clin. Sci.* 15, 361

WIDDOWSON E.M., McCANCE R.A. and SPRAY C.M. (1951) The chemical composition of the human body. *Clin. Sci.* 10, 113

WIGLEY R.D. (1960) Potassium deficiency in anorexia nervosa, with reference to renal tubular vacuolation. *Brit. med. J.* 2, 110

WILLIAMS R.T. (1963) Carcinoma of bronchus with hyponatraemia and dermatomyositis. *Brit. med. J.* 1, 233

WILKINSON A.W. (1960) *Body Fluids in Surgery*, 2nd edn. Edinburgh, 1960

WILLSON D.M., POWER M.H. and KEPLER E.J. (1940) Alkalosis and low potassium in a case of Cushing's syndrome: metabolic study. *J. clin. Invest.* 19, 701

★ WILSON G.M. (1963) Diuretics. *Brit. med. J.* 1, 285

WILSON G.M., OLNEY J.M., BROOKS L., MYRDEN J.A., BALL M.R. and MOORE F.D. (1954) Body sodium and potassium. II. A comparison of metabolic balance and isotope dilution methods of study. *Metabolism* 3, 324

WINKLER A.W., DANOWSKI T.S., ELKINTON J.R. and PETERS J.P. (1944) Electrolyte and fluid studies during water deprivation and starvation in human subjects, and effects of ingestion of fish, of carbohydrate, and of salt solutions. *J. clin. Invest.* 23, 807

WINTERS R.W., SCAGLIONE P.R., NAHAS G.G. and VEROSKY M. (1964) The mechanism of acidosis produced by hyperosmotic infusions. *J. clin. Invest.* 43, 647

WIRZ H., HARGITAY B. and KUHN W. (1951) Lokalisation des Konzentrierungsprozesses in der Niere durch direkte Kryoskopie. *Helv. physiol. pharmacol. acta.* 9, 196

WITTS L.J. (1937) Ritual purgation in modern medicine. *Lancet* 1, 427

★ WOLF A.V. (1958) *Thirst; Physiology of the Urge to Drink, and Problems of Water Lack.* Springfield, 1958

WOLFF H.P., KOCZOREK K.R. and BUCHBORN E. (1957) Hyperaldosteronism in heart disease. *Lancet* 2, 63

WOLFF H.P. and TORBICA M. (1963) Determination of plasma-aldosterone. *Lancet*, 1, 1346

★ WOOLMER R.F. (1959) *A symposium on pH and blood gas measurement.* Churchill, London, 1959

WOOTTON I.D.P. and KING E.J. (1953) Normal values for blood constituents. *Lancet* 1, 470

WRONG O. (1956) The relationship between water retention and electrolyte excretion following administration of anti-diuretic hormone. *Clin. Sci.* 15, 401

★ WRONG O. (1959) Sodium excretion and the control of extracellular fluid volume. *Lect. Scient. Basis Med.* 8, 386

WRONG O. (1962) Tests of renal function. Chapter 19 in *Renal Disease*, ed. D.A.K. Black, Blackwell, Oxford, 1962

WRONG O. and DAVIES H.E.F. (1959) The excretion of acid in renal disease. *Quart. J. Med.* **28,** 259

WRONG O., MORRISON R.B.I. and HURST P.E. (1961) A method of obtaining faecal fluid by *in vivo* dialysis. *Lancet* **1,** 1208

WYNN V. (1955) A metabolic study of acute water intoxication in man and dogs. *Clin. Sci.* **14,** 669

WYNN V. (1956) Water intoxication and serum hypotonicity. *Metabolism* **5,** 490

WYNN V. and HOUGHTON B.J. (1957) Observations in man upon the osmotic behaviour of the body cells after trauma. *Quart. J. Med.* **26,** 375

WYNN V. and ROB C.G. (1954) Water intoxication. *Lancet* **1,** 587

YAHR W.Z. and KRAKAUER J.S. (1965) Fluid requirements in Asiatic cholera. *Lancet* **1,** 1114

YATES F.E., URQUHART J. and HERBST A.L. (1958) Impairment of the enzymatic inactivation of adrenal cortical hormones following passive venous congestion of the liver. *Amer. J. Physiol.* **194,** 65

ZIERLER K.L. and ANDRES R. (1957) Movement of potassium into skeletal muscle during spontaneous attack in family periodic paralysis. *J. clin. Invest.* **36,** 730

ZIMMERMAN B., CASEY J.H. and BLOCH H.S. (1956) Mechanisms of sodium regulation in the surgical patient. *Surgery* **39,** 161

ZIMMERMAN B. and WANGENSTEEN O.H. (1952) Observations on water intoxication in surgical patients. *Surgery* **31,** 654

INDEX

Abortion, and hypernatraemia, 62
Acidosis, 68, 79, 92, 96
  clinical aspects, 118–21
  hydrion excess, 111–21
  metabolic, 112–14
  metabolic, lactic, 112, 113
  and potassium balance, 80
  renal, 114
    bicarbonate wastage, 114
    impaired excretion of ammonium, 115
    impaired excretion of titratable acid, 115
  respiratory, 116–18
  and sodium depletion, 50
Addison's disease, 42, 47, 51, 99, 100, 116
Adrenalectomy, 135
Adrenocorticotrophic hormone, 47
Albuminuria, 53, 96
Aldosterone, 64, 65, 66, 100
  antagonists, 72
  -secreting tumour, 96
  secretion rates in cardiac failure, 65
  and sodium balance, 44–46
Aldosteronism, primary and secondary, 65, 91, 93
Alimentary tract, electrolyte disturbances in, 136
  losses of K, 90
Alkalosis, 86, 93
  clinical aspects, 125–8
  contraction, 124
  hypokalaemic, 87, 129–30
  metabolic, 122–4
    renal response, 122
    respiratory response, 124
  and potassium balance, 80
  respiratory, 124–5

clinical cause, 127
and sodium depletion, 50
Aminoaciduria, 96
Aminophylline, 70
Ammonium, impaired excretion, 115
Angiotensin, 46, 48
Antidiuretic hormone, 23–25, 66, 96
  inappropriate secretion as cause of hyponatraemia, 58
  in water intoxication, 35
Antipyrine method, 2
Astrup apparatus, 107
Atrioventricular block, and potassium, 85

Bendrofluazide, 71
Bicarbonate, doses, 122
  plasma, laboratory investigations, 142
  wastage, 114
Body-fluid, see Fluid
Body water, total, 1
Bowel, ulceration, 71
Bronchial neoplasm, hyponatraemia in, 58
Bronchospasm, 120
Brönsted-Lowry terminology, 105–6

Capillary permeability, and oedema, 66–67
Carbon dioxide, elimination, daily, 123
  P_{CO_2}, 107–8, 116–17
  retention, 116
Cardiac arrest, 101–2, 120
  changes associated with hypokalaemia, 83, 101–2
  failure, 42, 64, 65
Cation exchange resins, 68
Cell metabolism, changes, 80–82
Cells, fluid components, 10

Cells, permeability and fluid components, 10, 18
transfer of K from, 101, 104
Chloride, and acid-base balance, 130-1
plasma, laboratory investigations, 142
Chlorothiazide, 71
Circulation, blood, electrolyte disturbances in, 137
Colonic washouts, 36
Congestive heart failure, 57, 64
Conn's syndrome, 65
Cortisone, 98
Cramps, 138
Cushing's disease, 17, 91

Dehydration, 28-37, 61
fever, 138
Desoxycorticosterone, 47
Deuterium method, 2
Diabetes insipidus, 71
of extrarenal origin, 26-27
nephrogenic, 27, 62
Diabetic coma, 79
hypernatraemia in, 61
Diarrhoea, 90, 95
as a cause of fluid loss, 50, 90, 95, 96
Diet, salt-free, 67-68
Digitalis, 84, 94, 95
Diuresis, antidiuretic hormone, 23
osmotic, 21, 22, 70
and sodium depletion, 52
water, 21
Diuretics, 19
Diurnal variation, 41, 42, 64, 77
Drowning, 36
Dyspnoea, paroxysmal nocturnal, 73

Electrolyte(s), disturbances, assessment, 132-4
general symptoms, 135
biological control, 14-18

relation to energy metabolism, 17
structure of the phases of body-fluid, 7-13
Electroneutrality, maintenance, 14
Enemata, 90
Energy and electrolytes, 17
Enteritis, staphylococcal, 51
Enzymes, and electrolyte concentration, 17
Ethacrynic acid, 72
Extracellular fluid, direct removal, 72
distribution, 3
plasma volume, 3, 14, 5
potassium concentration, 78
in tissue, 7
see also Electrolytes, Cells; Fluid, etc.

Faeces, potassium excretion, 77, 90
Fanconi syndrome, 93
Fibrocystic disease, and sodium depletion, 51
Fluid(s), balance, maintenance, 145
body, components, 5
comparison of intra- and extracellular components, 10
disorders and hydrion, 128-31
distribution, 3
distribution, osmotic determination, 14
electrolyte structure, 7-13
see also Extracellular fluid, Intracellular fluid
Frusemide, 73

Gastrectomy, 90
Gastro-enteritis, 94, 97
infantile, 90
Glomerular filtration rate, and potassium, 78
'Glomerular tubular imbalance', 43, 63

Glycosides, cardiac, 85

Heat effects, 41, 54, 62
Heart disease, and sodium excess, 64
see also Cardiac
Hydrion (Hydrogen ion), 105-31
  concentration, 107-8
  deficit, alkalosis, 121-8
  definition, 105
  excess, acidosis, 111-21
  homeostasis, 108-11
  plasma, laboratory investigations, 141
  relation to other disorders of body-
  fluid, 128-31
Hydrochlorothiazide, 71
Hydroflumethiazide, 71
Hypercapnia, 130
Hyperglycaemia, 16
Hyperkalaemia, 98-104
  action on heart, 101
  clinical spontaneous, 100
  prevention and treatment, 103
  see also Potassium
Hyperparathyroidism, 93
Hypernatraemia, and hypocalcaemia,
  62
  and salt poisoning, 61
  and water depletion, 60
Hypertension, malignant, and sodium
  depletion, 52
  and sodium balance, 48
Hyperventilation, 127
Hypoaldosteronism, 100, 101
Hypocalcaemia, and hypernatraemia, 62
Hypokalaemia, 83-86
  cardiac changes, 83
Hypokalaemic alkalosis, 129
Hyponatraemia, 16, 47, 72
  relative incidence of causes, 59
Hyponatraemic syndrome(s), 56-60
  classification, 56
Hypoproteinaemia, 66
Hyporolaemia, 72

Hypothermia, oedema after, 66

Infarction, myocardial, and potassium,
  85
Intracellular fluid, potassium content,
  77, 84
  in tissues, 7
  see also Electrolytes, Fluids, etc.
Intravenous feeding, 146

Kallikrein, 66
Kempner rice-fruit diet, 68
Kidneys, see Renal

Laboratory investigations, 139-45
Liquorice preparations, and potassium
  depletion, 91-92

Mannitol diuresis, 61
Mercurials, administration, 70-71
Metabolic acidosis, 112-14
Metabolic alkalosis, 122-4
Metabolism, energy, relation of electro-
  lytes to, 17
Metyrapone, 72
Micro-equivalents, ix
Milli-equivalents, ix
Muscles, electrolyte disturbances in, 137
  weakness, 85, 87
Myxoedema, 47

Natriuresis, 47, 48, 69
Necrosis, acute tubular, 63
  and sodium depletion, 52
Nephritis, acute, 63
Nephrotic syndrome, 63, 91
Nervous system, electrolyte distur-
  bances in, 137
Newborn, and K excess, 99
Norethisterone, 47

Oedema, 87, 99
  cardiac. 66

Oedema, episodic, 65
  generalized, and sodium excess, 60
  hepatic, 91
  and hypernatraemia, 62–72
  pre-menstrual, 47
  resistant, combination of agents, 72
Oliguria, 100
Osmolality, 14–17
  and thirst, 20

Palsy, familial periodic, 81, 82
Pancreas, islet-cell tumours, 90
Papillomata, colon and rectum, 90
Paralysis, 81, 82, 85, 103
  and potassium, 81–82
Peptic ulcer, 90
Plasma, K, 78–81
  laboratory investigations, 139–43
  Na, 54
  and respiratory acidosis, 118
  volume, in E.C.F., 3, 4, 5
  in water depletion, 33
Polydipsia, 26–27
Polyuria, 26–28, 51
Post-operative K depletion, 94
Potassium, administration, to muscle, 102
  of thiazides, 71
  amount and distribution, 74–76
  balance, external, 77
    changes, 79
  and changes in sodium balnace, 79
  depletion, 86–98
    clinical, 89–98
      alimentary losses of K, 89–90
      causes, 89
      picture and treatment, 93
      renal losses, 90
    experimental, 86–89
    symptoms, 85–86
  homeostasis, 76
  plasma, laboratory investigations,141
  in stored blood, 99

see also Hyperkalaemia, Hypokalae-
  mia
Progesterone, and sodium balance, 47
Propranolol, 64
Protein anabolism, and cellular uptake
  of K, 71
Protein-losing gastro-enteropathy, 66
Purgation, 90
  dangers, 57
Pyloric stenosis, 89

Renal acidosis, 114
  disease, intrinsic and sodium excess,
    63
  primary, and loss of K, 92
  failure, 103, 104
    chronic, and sodium depletion, 52–
      53
  losses of K, 90
  perfusion, inadequate, and sodium
    excess, 64
  tubular dysfunction, 93
Replacement therapy, 145, 147
Respiratory system, electrolyte disturbances in, 137
Rice diet, and sodium depletion, 53

Saline, hypertonic, 44, 55, 57
Salt depletion, iatrogenic, 57
  poisoning and hypernatraemia, 61
  treatment, 62
  see also Sodium
Serum C′1-esterase, 66
Simmonds' disease, 47
Skin rashes, 71
Sodium, amount and distribution, 39–
  40
  amount filtered at glomerulus, in-
    crease, 70
  balance, 40
    changes, 79
  depletion, 49–56
    causes, 49

Sodium, depletion—*contd.*
  clinical, 50
  definition, 49
  diagnosis, 54
  experimental studies, 49
  symptoms, 50
  treatment, 55
  and water intoxication, 35
 excess, 60–73
  treatment, 67
   increase of urinary sodium output, 69
   restriction of intake, 67
  homeostasis, 40
  hyponatraemic syndromes, 56–60
  lactate, 121
  plasma, laboratory investigations, 140
  reabsorption, excessive, 64–67
  renal handling, 42
  in stools, 51
  turnover, 48
Southey's tubes, 73
Spirolactones, 72
Steatorrhoea, 17, 90
Sweat, cause of sodium depletion, 51
  potassium loss in, 77
  water loss, 1

Tachycardia, paroxysmal atrial, with variable atrioventricular block, (P.A.T.B.), 84, 94, 95
Tetany, 85, 87, 126
THAM, 121
Thiazides, 116
  administration, 71
Thirst, 19
  and antidiuretic hormone, 23–25
  centre, 21
  physiology, 20
  and urinary concentration and dilution, 21
Thrombocytopenia, 71
Tissue damage in K depletion, 88

electrolytes, 7, 8
Treatment, 132–50
  history and examination, 135–9
  laboratory investigations, 139–45
  principles, 145–50
  see also Sodium; Potassium, etc.
Tuberculosis, 59
Tubular transport, active, inhibitors, 70

Ulcerative colitis, 17, 90
Uraemia, 126
  extrarenal, and sodium depletion, 53
Urea, blood, 16, 52, 54
Urinary system, electrolyte disturbances in, 136
Urine, concentration, and dilution, and thirst, 21
  laboratory investigations, 144
  output of K, 86
  Na output, 43, 44, 51
  in water depletion, 32

Voice, in electrolyte imbalance, 138
Vomiting, 95
  and losses of K, 89

Water, balance, 19
  body, 19–38
  and polyuria, 26–28
  depletion, 28–37, 91
   clinical, 30
   diagnosis, 32
   experimental, 28
   treatment, 33
  drinking, compulsive, 26
  intoxication, 34–38
   diagnosis, 35, 37
   and patient's own discretion, 36
   post-operative, 36
   symptoms, 36
  requirements, 31
  see also Body-water; Fluids, etc.